Praise for *Fertility Rules*

"So much more than the birds and the bees! Leslie Schrock demystifies human reproduction in her meticulously researched *Fertility Rules*. Written in a way readers can understand, she breaks down the latest data behind fertility, infertility, and miscarriage. Essential reading for those wanting to understand how their body works, improve chances of conception, and take a deep dive into the facts."
　　　　—Dana McQueen, MD, MAS, reproductive endocrinologist

"*Fertility Rules* provides an excellent education in reproductive physiology, conception, and infertility for anyone on the fertility journey or will be one day. Personal vignettes and a friendly tone help make the topics approachable and provide meaningful suggestions for men or women about achieving reproductive health."
　　　　—Michael L. Eisenberg, MD, director of male reproductive medicine and surgery, Stanford University School of Medicine

"Air pollution and plastics are warming our planet. Who knew it was harming our fertility too? *Fertility Rules* is the trusted companion everyone should have. Leslie Schrock weaves science with real talk. This book gives you the confidence to navigate your fertility journey."
　　　　—Ryan Panchadsaram, coauthor of *Speed and Scale*

Praise for *Bumpin'* by Leslie Schrock

2020 National Parenting Award Winner

"A smart, approachable guide packed with practical advice for parents who want a science-backed, individualized approach to pregnancy."
—Linda Avey, cofounder of 23andMe

"We are leading our lives with more intention than ever before and want to make informed choices based on research from people we trust. Leslie has distilled everything you need to know about pregnancy in one place in a warm, approachable way so you can feel confident, informed, and excited to make this important journey your own."
—Jessica Rolph, cofounder and CEO of Lovevery

"Pregnancy can be a scary and confusing time with conflicting information coming from everyone you know. . . . *Bumpin'* by Leslie Schrock is a wonderful companion for moms-to-be. It covers it all, from eggs, ovulation, and sex to pregnancy-friendly exercises and post-delivery recovery. It's like chatting with your best pal, who happens to be super knowledgeable."
—Elena Epstein, director of the National Parenting Product Awards

fertility rules

Also by Leslie Schrock

Bumpin': The Modern Guide to Pregnancy

fertility rules

The Definitive Guide to Male and Female Reproductive Health

leslie schrock

Medical editor: Jane van Dis, MD: Obstetrics/Gynecology

Scientific editor: Christopher De Jonge, PhD, HCLD (ABB): Urology/Andrology

Expert contributors: Michaela Burns, Women's Health Physical Trainer
Aliza Marogy, Registered Nutritionist, Naturopathic Doctor
Liz Miracle, PT, MSPT, Women's Health Clinical Specialist

Simon Element

New York   London   Toronto   Sydney   New Delhi

**SIMON
ELEMENT**

An Imprint of Simon & Schuster, Inc.
1230 Avenue of the Americas
New York, NY 10020

First Simon Element trade paperback edition June 2023

SIMON ELEMENT is a trademark of Simon & Schuster, Inc.

For information about special discounts for bulk purchases, please contact
Simon & Schuster Special Sales at 1-866-506-1949 or business@simonandschuster.com.

The Simon & Schuster Speakers Bureau can bring authors to your live event.
For more information or to book an event, contact the Simon & Schuster Speakers
Bureau at 1-866-248-3049 or visit our website at www.simonspeakers.com.

Interior design by Lexy East

Manufactured in the United States of America

10 9 8 7 6 5 4 3 2 1

Library of Congress Cataloging-in-Publication Data has been applied for.

ISBN 978-1-6680-0014-4
ISBN 978-1-6680-0015-1 (ebook)

To my boys,
TJ and Dylan

We cannot direct the wind, but we can adjust the sails.

—Dolly Parton

CONTENTS

fertility
rules

INTRODUCTION

Like so many couples in our thirties, my husband, Nick, and I assumed having a baby would be easy. Because, really, how hard could it be? We've all heard the story of the single celebrity who welcomed a baby at fifty-one, or know a friend who got surprise pregnant at forty-three, or the couple who tried to conceive for years and finally did after they "just relaxed."

After three miscarriages, two sons, tests, and conversations with fertility experts around the world, we still don't have a diagnosis beyond "bad luck." And I am not the only one. After writing my first book, *Bumpin'*, I heard similar stories from readers who also spent long hours analyzing what they could have done differently. Finding the answer to that question led me on a yearslong quest to assemble everything I wish I'd known about fertility before trying to conceive. The culmination of that pursuit is the book in your hands.

No one thinks much about their fertility until they have to. But for many of us, that's already too late. At least one in six couples struggle to conceive. Sperm concentration and total count have dropped more than 50 percent since the 1970s, and no one really understands why. Miscarriages, diminished ovarian reserves, and disorders like polycystic ovary syndrome (PCOS) and endometriosis are on the rise, and 13 percent of women cannot get or stay pregnant. Endocrine-disrupting chemicals (EDC) in the environment and at home are interfering with our hormones, hurting fertility and future pregnancies, and cascading into chronic health conditions like diabetes and obesity. And we don't have simple solutions to deal with any of this. What we do have is a cottage industry of wellness influencers recommending expensive fertility supplements, special diets, and plans that are rarely supported by research and have little impact on true medical conditions. Fertility treatments are also exorbitantly priced and geographically inaccessible for most people. And even though around half of infertility is due to problems in men's bodies, all of this is marketed to women, as the culture of fertility is and has always been female.

Women are told, often and repeatedly by friends, family, the fertility industry, the media, and strangers that their fertile years slip toward zero after thirty-five. Women are told they are selfish for waiting to have a baby, the assumption being it's about work rather than the more common reason: they cannot find a partner. Women's lifestyle choices—what they eat, drink, and use on their bodies—are scrutinized and judged, before conception through pregnancy and into the postpartum period. But men experience age-related fertility decline too, and sperm is influenced by the same lifestyle factors. Unlike eggs, which once abnormal cannot be fixed, sperm regenerate constantly and can be improved. Yet men are rarely told how. And who would tell them?

Our only body education today is fear and abstinence. Remember the sex-ed demonstration by the school nurse, or the adolescent rite of passage aka "the talk"? Both cover the same concepts—birth control, saying no to sex, avoiding pregnancy, and STDs—but little else about how our bodies work. Armed with a box of tampons (and more questions than answers), girls are left to figure out their periods on their own. Half of adult women—including medical school students—don't know what or when ovulation is or any other basics of their menstrual cycles. For boys, sperm and reproductive health remain a mystery into adulthood, and men believe if they can ejaculate they can make a baby, which isn't always the case.

The healthcare system isn't working particularly well for anyone either. Women's routine health checks consist of quick chats with a gynecologist about preventing or enabling pregnancy, a pelvic exam, and a Pap smear every few years until they decide to conceive. Once they are pregnant, it's too late to do much about underlying conditions that can cause complications. While urology deals with the urinary tract and andrology addresses infertility, there is no specialty focused solely on male reproductive health as gynecology does for women.

Men are poor utilizers of healthcare in general. Some 41 percent of US men report that they were told as children that men don't complain or talk about their health issues. Three out of four men would rather mow the lawn or go shopping with their partner than go to the doctor. And twenty-five percent of men are never even examined during infertility explorations. Ultimately, this leaves women to serve as treatment surrogates for men, undergoing lengthy, invasive, expensive, and in some cases unnecessary procedures when all that may be required is for their partner to get a semen analysis, have a physical exam, and make basic lifestyle tweaks.

The bulk of today's medical research and guidance is based upon the study of men's bodies. But there is one area where this is not the case. Though our dismal maternal health outcomes do not reflect it, men's reproductive health is even less understood than women's. Sperm is a biomarker for a man's overall health, and abnormal levels can indicate serious health problems like tumors, cancer, diabetes, and overall morbidity and mortality. Since men's life spans are already five years shorter than women's and dropping, a simple semen analysis could become a diagnostic tool used to extend or even save lives. However, we still live in a world where the word *sperm* is banned on most ad platforms (as are *uterus* and *vagina*) and is rarely (if ever) uttered aloud to a loved one or anyone else. Until this topic is destigmatized, men will suffer from avoidable chronic conditions and early death, and women and families will suffer right along with them. On a personal note, I am now a mother to two young boys. Seeing what is going on in men's health fills me with dread for them, and this book was written with their futures in mind. But I am hopeful that things may be changing.

When I started working in health tech over a decade ago, the ecosystem of apps, tests, and gadgets to manage and teach reproductive health was in its infancy. Now it's one of the fastest-growing areas of healthcare, and as one of the most active investors and advisers in the space, I'm right at the center of it. Consumer technology companies are transforming how and where we take care of our bodies, with more convenient options available from anywhere—not just the doctor's office. From telemedicine appointments with experts around the world for a second opinion to at-home hormone and semen testing and AI-powered birth control, technology has changed not only what's possible but also our ability to understand and translate what's happening inside of our bodies in real time. A surge of new research, methods, technologies, and techniques to help couples struggling to conceive are emerging too. Machine-learning models are improving the in vitro fertilization (IVF) process, from optimizing egg retrieval to determining when to deliver a trigger shot and selecting the best quality embryo. More precise at-home tests combine luteinizing hormone (LH) surge data with progesterone levels to better pinpoint the fertile window and ensure that women are ovulating when they think they are.

As far as we've come, today's tests and treatments have limits that the fertility industry does not communicate clearly. At-home hormone screenings for biomarkers like anti-Mullerian hormone (AMH) can lead women to believe they will have trouble conceiving when in fact, AMH is not a good single indicator of overall fertility or the ability to get pregnant naturally. Egg freezing is marketed as an insurance policy for women waiting to start a family. But when it comes time to unfreeze, there is no guarantee there will be a baby down the road. With egg freezing, the only information you have post-retrieval is how many are on ice; there is no way to test the quality of a single egg. Once eggs are fertilized, many will not survive. Those who genetically test the embryos that survive five days to become blastocysts may then find that a high percentage are abnormal.

ART is shorthand for assisted reproduction technology, and providers often refer to their work as more of an art than a science. In an industry as data- and research-driven as medicine, this statement is mind-boggling. But I discovered interviewing specialists across the globe that it's accurate. There are not industry-wide best practices for many procedures and treatments are highly bespoke depending upon the clinic and provider you choose.

WHAT YOU'RE ABOUT TO READ

After years of research and hundreds of conversations with founders, doctors, and health experts, *Fertility Rules* parses everything we know—and what we don't—about female and male fertility. Mixing clinical data with a bit of history, the latest technology, and practical advice, it provides tools to manage and understand your fertility. It exposes misinformation and debunks the most common false assumptions medical professionals hear from patients. Myths like:

- Birth control hurts fertility. (Birth control has no long-term effect on fertility, though some types delay its return.)
- A normal period regardless of age means getting pregnant is a guarantee. (There are many factors— underlying health conditions, medications, and egg and sperm quality—that influence the ability to get and stay pregnant.)
- Because I'm healthy, my ovaries and eggs will be too—even though I'm over forty. (There will be fewer chromosomally normal eggs after forty no matter what you do or how healthy you are.)
- Diet greatly impacts egg quality. (Diet is important to your overall fertility, but cannot fix chromosomally abnormal eggs.)

- Every pregnancy results in a live birth. (It does not.)
- It takes only one sperm to make a baby, so fertility isn't a man's problem. (Sperm is half the genetic basis of a human, and problems in men's bodies are the cause of around half of all infertility.)

Here is another truth that all medical professionals wish their patients knew: fertility doesn't just magically improve after eating blueberries or taking coenzyme Q10 (CoQ10) for a few weeks (although do that—they're great!) or cleansing. "Just relaxing" isn't a thing either, and please never say that to someone who is having trouble conceiving. Optimizing fertility is a full-body commitment to a healthier lifestyle. Eating well, exercising, and stopping behaviors like smoking, cannabis, and drinking before trying to conceive are good for your health no matter what. But all the good habits in the world cannot overcome medical conditions like blocked fallopian tubes or azoospermia, and babies are not handed out on a merit system. From managing your mental health (stress-induced cortisol is a fertility killer) to eating a diet packed with whole foods (processed foods, trans fats, and added sugar are not fertility-friendly) to finding a physical activity you enjoy (it doesn't have to be yoga) and taking supplements if appropriate (while understanding how serious their effects can be), improving lifestyle factors gives your body the best possible shot.

Fertility Rules is split into three parts:

1. Setting a baseline: Understanding your body and your partner's and all of the fertility basics.
2. Optimizing male and female fertility: Identifying and tweaking the most important lifestyle factors.
3. Taking action: How making a baby really works; fertility testing; egg, sperm, and embryo freezing; and treatment options if you run into challenges.

WHO SHOULD READ THIS BOOK?

If you flipped through the table of contents and thought it was written exclusively for people thinking about or actively trying to get pregnant, what I'm about to say may come as a surprise. Though I expect most readers will pick this book up for that purpose, there is so much more to fertility than making babies. Fertility is a mirror of your overall health, from adolescence through menopause. Or manopause, which, yep, is a real thing. On that note, even though I know that women are the more likely readers, this book is written for men too, so share it with your partner, son, friend, brother, and anyone else you care about.

THE DATA

Male fertility is underfunded relative to other medical issues, and as a result, we know very little beyond the basics. Women of reproductive age were excluded from clinical trials for decades, and even today, women are not well represented, especially women of color. Fertility research suffers from a dearth of equal representation across gender, racial, and cultural groups, a lack of funding and interest from researchers, and confounding factors that can be difficult to unravel. Our current body of fertility data is also sourced mostly from studies of assisted reproduction, not natural conception.

Even as demand grows and new and better technologies launch, IVF outcomes are declining globally and assisted reproduction is and always has been a sticky topic in the research community. The first scientist to successfully perform intrauterine insemination (IUI) with donor sperm in 1953 was told inseminating women with sperm that was not their husband's was "contrary to public policy and good morals," so that accomplishment was a closely guarded secret for a decade. The scientists who brought forth the first IVF baby, in 1978, were denied public funding for their research on moral grounds, and the patriarch of Venice claimed that artificial insemination would lead to women being used as "baby factories." The Catholic Church criticized semen donors as adulterers who promoted the vice of masturbation and claimed that the practice encouraged eugenic government policies. Assisted reproduction and technologies like polygenic risk scores are still condemned as a disguise for eugenics. Even amidst the controversy, compelling research is underway and there are guidelines everyone can follow. This book gives an overview of evidence-backed ways to understand and improve your fertility. However, it is not Wikipedia and cannot capture every single condition. If you do read about an issue and think, *That's me*, skip Dr. Google and call a physician, as your care should be individualized. For research wonks or those looking for a deeper look into a specific topic, flip to the back and explore the endnotes. A glossary of terms and abbreviations is also there since there are so many to remember.

SEEKING CARE

Finding help can be complicated, and many men still power through healthcare needs (but seriously, guys, please stop avoiding medical care!). For women, especially women of color, medical gaslighting (feeling trivialized or dismissed by medical providers, or having your condition blamed on mental illness) ends in mostly preventable diagnostic errors, which happen in up to one in seven clinical encounters. Women are misdiagnosed more frequently than men, and their health problems are often blamed on mental health struggles. Many women describe being treated differently than men or feeling ignored when they do seek help. Today's high-stress medical culture makes this dynamic worse. Even before the pandemic, health professionals from all specialties reported record levels of burnout. Doctor's visits should be longer, but because they work under difficult, stressful conditions and there is a shortage of medical providers in general, they are forced to take on more patients than is optimal.

The result is patients feel rushed, and because there is a lack of trust in these relationships, they are more likely to lie if they feel ashamed, especially when answering questions about their number of sexual partners or alcohol consumption. But doctors cannot do their jobs without the truth, as small pieces of information can be important. So, be honest in appointments—there is nothing they haven't heard before.

Asking questions is critical when navigating fertility treatment. My hope is that walking into an appointment with the knowledge in this book grows the confidence required to advocate for yourself there and in all other healthcare settings. There is a whole section dedicated to choosing a fertility clinic if you do encounter issues and questions to ask during a provider interview in chapter 14. If you have a relationship with a medical professional who makes you feel invisible, ignored, marginalized, or worse, it's time to find someone else. If you have no choice but to see that person, take a friend, partner, or family member to your appointment. They can be the official notetaker and provide a third-party point of view that may help with treatment and diagnosis. As a patient, it is your right to ask as many questions as you'd like for as long as your appointment allows. Informed consent is at the center of all medical relationships and means understanding and giving an okay to what is being done to you, including all treatments.

A FINAL NOTE BEFORE WE START

Our healthcare system only knows how to treat disease when it's already present and diagnosed correctly. Beyond helping you improve your fertility I want to put you into a preventive mindset to avoid problems before they happen. We have a tremendous amount of work to do, and the healthcare system cannot do everything for us. We must understand and take responsibility for our own bodies, make decisions, and act. My ambitious hope is that awareness will also drive more funding into fertility research, open conversation about infertility, shut down the influencers who are cheating desperate patients out of thousands of dollars, make us take a hard look at what we're eating, and that everyone will have more answers and options in the future.

Putting this book in front of men and women is why there are two medical and scientific editors: one for women's health and one for men's. Jane van Dis, MD, and Christopher De Jonge, PhD, are experienced and exceptionally curious and passionate clinicians and researchers, with a combined five decades of practice. They vetted all studies, research, and medical guidelines.

The intersection of gender identity and healthcare is complex, and gender-affirming care is critical. For up-to-date resources including patient rights, visit the National Center for Transgender Equality at www.transequality.org, GLAAD at www.glaad.org, or Family Equality www.familyequality.org. For purposes of simplicity, this book uses pronouns coded for the cisgender experience.

Why, hello there. These sections appear throughout to recount my fertility journey and personal commentary separately from the science. If a similarly complex experience brings you here, know that you are not alone, and there are evidence-backed ways to improve your odds. If you're just starting out or are reading because you are fertility curious, sharing my story is not meant to cause anxiety. Even if you have an easy time, someone in your life will not, so it's useful to understand the spectrum of experiences.

Part 1

What You May
Not Know

Chapter 1

THE MENSTRUAL CYCLE

Your cycle is a vital sign—and the simplest
way to understand female fertility

In 1985, a twenty-one-year-old Courteney Cox shattered taboos by uttering the word period in a Tampax commercial. Even though half of humans have one, that ad marked the first time that word was heard on television. We've come a long way since, but one in four UK women don't understand their cycle, over half of American women feel embarrassed while it's happening, and 62 percent also claim their period-related pain was not taken seriously by doctors. The menstrual cycle's mysterious status is a big problem, as it is the best real-time indicator of a woman's overall health and fertility. It is a vital sign just like temperature that gives rise to different moods, energy, sexual desire, and brain function. Many women live with symptoms that are considered "normal"—like cramps—that can indicate underlying health issues. In many cases, these symptoms and conditions are treatable or even preventable—if you know what to do about it. Understanding when you ovulate and the fertile window are the most critical pieces of data if you're trying to conceive (TTC) too. Yet discussion of any of these topics (much less a basic education) happens privately, if at all, which is why we're starting at the beginning, so you know what's normal and what's not.

Whether you call it the red wave, Auntie Flo, monthly friend, red wedding, chum, girl flu, shark week, red panda, or another questionable nickname, your period is not the whole menstrual cycle—it's just the first part. The menstrual cycle is actually two separate cycles: one that happens in your uterus and another in your ovaries. Ovulation, the release of a mature egg, is common to both cycles and happens at the same time midway through. The menstrual cycle's purpose each month is to diligently prepare a hospitable home in the uterus for a future fetus and then discard that home if it isn't needed. The period happens each month when a woman's body jettisons the uterine lining it prepared for a potential pregnancy. It is triggered by the fall in estrogen and progesterone levels that occurs when you are not pregnant, and the discarded uterine lining is the source of blood. The first period arrives when girls hit puberty, around ten or eleven years old, in an event called menarche, and ends for good during menopause, between ages forty-five and fifty-five.

So you can visualize where all of this happens, here is an internal view of the female reproductive system. Notice that the line to the vagina is not pointing to the outside. That's correct: the vagina is on the *inside* of your body. The outer part of female genitalia is called the vulva and includes the opening to the vagina, the labia majora (outer lips), the labia minora (inner lips), and the clitoris.

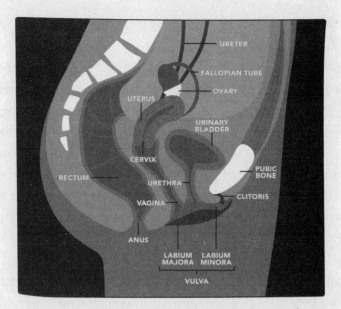

MENSTRUAL CYCLE PHASES

Using a generic twenty-eight-day cycle as a template, the pre-ovulation phase, which includes your period, happens between cycle days one and fourteen. Ovulation takes place between cycle days fourteen and sixteen, and the post-ovulation phase lasts until your next period begins.

	Pre-ovulation (Days 1-14)		Ovulation (Days 14-16)	Post-ovulation (Days 16-28)
Ovarian cycle	Follicular phase			Luteal phase
Uterine cycle	Period	Proliferative phase		Secretory phase

Ovarian cycle

Follicular phase: The days between the start of your period and ovulation. Estrogen rises as your ovarian follicles develop to nurture the immature eggs that may be released during ovulation. Think of these follicles as tiny nests within the ovaries. Your pituitary gland produces luteinizing hormone (LH) during this time, which signals the ovaries to ovulate or release the mature egg. Energy levels will be high, your sex drive may rise as you approach ovulation, and skin quality is at its best.

Luteal phase: The time from ovulation to the start of your next period when your body prepares for a possible pregnancy. The follicle that released the egg turns into a hormone-producing center called the corpus luteum (a cyst on your ovary that alerts the uterus to prepare for a possible pregnancy) and starts to produce progesterone and estrogen. These hormone changes cause PMS symptoms like headaches, bloating, acne, and mood shifts. Expect to be more tired during the luteal phase, and for your immune response to be lower too.

Ovulation

Bisecting both the uterine and ovarian cycles, ovulation is the midcycle release of the mature egg from its follicle. Lasting between twelve to twenty-four hours, estrogen peaks and along with it your energy. Your libido may be higher, and it is the most fertile time of your cycle, when you are most likely to get pregnant.

Uterine cycle

Period: Your period does not punctuate the end of your cycle; it marks the beginning. It happens when your body sheds the uterine lining it doesn't need for pregnancy through your cervix (think of the cervix as the door to your uterus) and out of your vagina. During this phase, estrogen and progesterone levels are low. Expect energy dips, keep things mellow, do a little self-care, and keep exercise gentle.

Proliferative phase: The time between the end of your period and ovulation when your uterus rebuilds that embryo-friendly lining. The lining of the uterus becomes thick and spongy as it expands to ready itself for a possible pregnancy. The cervix goes through changes too, dilating and producing a watery mucous discharge that makes the vagina less acidic, making it easier for sperm to enter.

Secretory phase: In a twenty-eight-day cycle, this phase occurs between days fourteen and twenty-eight. Progesterone levels rise at the beginning of this phase, and the endometrium becomes its thickest, cushiest version so a fertilized egg can burrow in. If an egg is not fertilized, the uterine lining breaks down and is shed during your period.

. . . .

Your brain functions differently through each menstrual cycle phase too. The hormones that trigger the change between fertile and infertile days affect the hippocampus, your regulator of emotions and memory. The hippocampus changes visually as ovarian hormone levels fluctuate, and changing sex hormone levels impact the network properties of the cerebellum, the seat of motor skills and human learning, memory, and decision-making. How does this manifest? The follicular phase is associated with better spatial skills but more anxiety. Toward ovulation, your imagination may improve along with perception, memory, and social abilities. Sexual desire peaks at ovulation, then things get more mellow as you enter the luteal phase, which is all about calm, chill vibes.

MENSTRUAL CYCLE FAQS

How do I know if my menstrual cycle is normal?

A textbook cycle is between twenty-one and thirty-eight days long. It has a consistent duration month to month, with bleeding for between four and seven days. Normal menstrual fluid is bright red like cranberry juice and free of clots, though at the beginning or the end of your period, blood may be dark or brown. Volume-wise, filling up a tampon, pad, or cup every four hours is considered normal. Bleeding between cycles is considered abnormal. Irregular or abnormal cycles can indicate fertility problems or conditions like polycystic ovarian syndrome (PCOS) or amenorrhea (the absence of a period), so if you notice yours is off, take notes and book an appointment with your gynecologist.

How long is the typical menstrual cycle?

We throw around twenty-eight days as the standard, but just 13 percent of women have a twenty-eight-day cycle. Every woman's cycle is different and can change over time. A cycle duration outside of twenty-one to thirty-eight days is considered atypical, and consistency from cycle to cycle matters more than the length if it is in that zone. If it's thirty-one days one month and twenty-four the next, that is an irregular cycle.

How do I figure out my cycle length?

The first day of your period is day one, and the number of days until it begins again is your cycle length. So, to determine how long yours is, start counting on the day your period arrives (that's day one) and stop the day before it restarts.

Why should I track my period?

Period details are helpful when dealing with a new symptom or if you need a record of your cycle for conception purposes. With enough historical data, period-tracking apps can raise your chances of conception by 20 percent each cycle. The key is using them a few months in advance of trying to conceive so there is enough data for the app's algorithms to project an accurate fertile window. Cycle trackers ask for a range of data, like the date your period started, how long it lasted, symptoms, volume, color, sleep quality, exercise, and stress. Some apps integrate data from sensors and devices that passively track activity and sleep too. One other bonus of cycle tracking: if you do get pregnant, the first day of the last menstrual period (known as LMP) is what ob-gyns use to calculate a due date. This is useful since half of women cannot recall LMP during their first prenatal appointment. If you do use an app or platform that stores your data, read the terms and conditions. It is wise to ensure the company anonymizes its user data and will not share it. If you aren't comfortable using an app, a normal calendar or planner is fine too.

How do I know if I'm ovulating?

Measuring your basal body temperature (BBT—it rises during ovulation), tracking changes in your cervix or cervical mucus (you're looking for a slippery, egg white consistency), or looking for the luteinizing hormone (LH) surge twenty-four to thirty-six hours pre-ovulation using urine tests are the main ways to track ovulation. After you release an egg, your progesterone levels will be higher, but the rise only means that you ovulated recently, not whether you will again or if it's happening now. Measuring a rise in progesterone right after ovulation or getting a positive pregnancy test are the only two ways to know for sure that you truly ovulated. Today's basic drugstore ovulation-predictor kits (OPKs) test for the presence of LH in urine while more sophisticated versions identify the rise in progesterone too. Some people have changes in libido around ovulation (as in it's raging) or experience light cramping. But a few notes on OPKs: the LH surge is a sign your body is trying to ovulate, not a signal that it released an egg—only progesterone or two pink lines can tell you that. If you have a short surge and only check once per day, or your peak LH levels are below what the test can detect, OPKs may not work for you. Women with PCOS can have high LH levels constantly or intermittently, which means OPKs can stay positive even if you're not ovulating. Fertility drugs, hormone therapies, and antibiotics that include tetracycline can interfere with OPK effectiveness too. If you have cycle-related conditions, it is useful to try multiple methods, like using BBT in combination with OPKs, to best identify your fertile window. If you're period tracking, your app's algorithm will send you a notification when it thinks your fertile window begins and when you'll ovulate next.

How much blood do I lose during my period?

Although it looks like a lot, the amount of blood eliminated by your body during your period is just two to four tablespoons. Menstrual fluid isn't just blood—it also contains a mix of mucus, tissue, and the uterine lining your body no longer needs.

Does a heavy period mean there is something wrong?

Not necessarily. But consistently heavy periods can be signs of underlying health conditions like PCOS, thyroid problems, and precancerous growths, or side effects of medications like an intrauterine device (IUD) that can cause longer, heavier, irregular cycles, or lifestyle factors that cause hormone imbalances. To gauge if it's too much bleeding, look at the volume markings on your menstrual cup or pay attention to how long it takes to soak through pads and tampons. If you're soaking through a super absorbent pad or tampon or filling a cup faster than one to two hours, bleed heavily for longer than seven days, or pass blood clots that are larger than a quarter, talk to your doctor. Volume can change from month to month, so unless it's an extreme amount, evaluate it over several cycles.

What if I don't have a period? Is that bad?

Amenorrhea, or the absence of a period, is not always a reason to panic. If you've had a period and it suddenly vanishes, though, pay attention. Stress can play a factor, as can strenuous exercise, and women who are more than 10 percent underweight often experience longer-term amenorrhea. There are also forms of birth control that eliminate your period, and medications that treat high blood pressure and allergies can impact its presence too. A missing period can be an early indicator of premature menopause or indicate hormonal imbalances like PCOS and thyroid problems. If your period stops for more than six months, make an appointment with your gynecologist or primary care doctor. Rarely, it can be a sign of dysplasia or precancer in the uterus, and that requires immediate treatment.

Which period products are the most fertility-friendly?

When it comes to choosing the best period products to optimize your fertility, which one is right is a matter of weighing their pros and cons against your period and lifestyle. But none of today's options negatively impact your fertility. If that surprises you, you're probably thinking of a condition associated with tampons. Toxic shock syndrome (TSS) is caused by the presence of staph or strep bacteria, with symptoms including a high fever (over 102 degrees Fahrenheit), vomiting, rash, and sore throat. TSS happens to women whose immune systems do not produce sufficient antibody responses to the toxins produced by the bacteria. TSS nearly put a halt to the tampon's rising popularity in the 1970s and 1980s after a rash of cases were linked to a brand no longer on the market. While tampons are a risk factor for TSS, more than half of today's cases are unrelated to menstruation. The other negative association with tampons is that trace amounts of dioxin, a pollutant linked to hormone disruption and cancer, were detected in previous versions. Dioxin levels in today's tampons are 13,000 to 240,000 times less than dietary exposures. Tampons are Class II FDA-regulated medical devices to ensure they are constructed of safe materials and marketed correctly. While pads and tampons still dominate the market, new period-management solutions put more focus on comfort, reusability, sustainability, and empowerment. Period discs and cups are reusable and inserted into the vagina to catch period blood up to twelve hours. Period underwear is indetectable and looks completely normal and (dare I say) cute.

What other health problems can my cycle trigger?

Hormone fluctuations during different menstrual cycle phases can create chaos for many of the body's systems. From irritable bowel syndrome (IBS), which causes bloating, gas, and cramping right before your period starts, to cramps caused by bladder pain, menstrual migraines, and depression and anxiety that visit along with your period, symptoms usually pop up before or during cycle resets each month. These health problems can be indicative of an underlying condition or side effects of lifestyle factors. Pending how serious they are, it is worth a chat with your favorite provider if they disrupt your quality of life or worsen over time.

What happens to my period as I age?

At the start of your fertile years during menarche, periods are heavier and can be longer. Three years after menarche, they tend to even out and become more regular through your twenties and thirties. Then in your forties, as your body transitions through perimenopause into menopause, cycles are more irregular, lighter, or heavier than usual, or stop and start at random. And an average of forty years after they began, your period stops entirely, between the ages of forty-five and fifty-five.

Pause . . . WTF is perimenopause?

Ah yes, the entrée to menopause that most people have never heard of. Literally meaning "around menopause," perimenopause can start in your thirties but on average occurs between ages forty and forty-four. The dip in your body's production of estrogen and progesterone is responsible for these changes, which include hot flashes, night sweats, mood swings, changes to libido, vaginal dryness, weight gain, issues with bone density, heightened PMS, and irregular cycles. So how do you know if you're experiencing perimenopause? If there are sixty days or more between cycles, or your cycle consistently shifts by seven days or more each time, that's one sign. There are blood tests that measure the three hormones that change with perimenopause—estradiol, FSH, and LH—available to order from consumer-testing companies too.

Hold on, that sounds like menopause. So, what's the difference?

There are three stages to the menopause journey that conclude your fertile years. Perimenopause is the time leading up to menopause, and you'll likely still have some periods, though they will become irregular. Menopause shares all of perimenopause's wild symptoms and can last for up to a decade, though periods will become less and less frequent. Postmenopause describes the time after at least twelve months have gone by with no period and all menopause symptoms eventually fade away. Unlike the media portrayal, your sex life isn't over when you hit this life phase; your vagina does not dry out, and there is no requirement that you sport a Golden Girls coiffure. Many women report that they enjoy sex (and their lives in general) more after menopause because they don't have to worry about getting pregnant and love the freedom from mercurial hormonal symptoms.

COMMON GYNECOLOGICAL CONDITIONS THAT CAN BE GATEWAYS TO SUBFERTILITY OR INFERTILITY

One in five women is affected by endometriosis or PCOS during their reproductive years, and there is no definitive test to diagnose either condition. The result is that the average time from onset of symptoms to diagnosis for both is more than ten years, and like the other

Condition	What is it?	Symptoms	
Amenorrhea	The lack of a period, which often results in anovulation.	Missing period sometimes accompanied by a headache or vision changes, nausea, extra facial hair or hair loss, changes in breast size, stretch marks, and breast discharge.	
Bacterial vaginosis (BV)	An overgrowth of bad bacteria in the vagina that can affect IVF outcomes.	It is asymptomatic 84 percent of the time, but symptoms can include itching, burning when peeing, odor, or abnormal vaginal discharge.	

conditions here, they impact your fertility. If any of these symptoms are familiar, schedule an appointment with your gynecologist or primary care provider, especially if conception is on your mind. Dr. Google is not your friend—there is a lot of conflicting information out there—so try to keep your search activity to a minimum.

	Causes	Treatment
	Primary amenorrhea is caused by genetic and chromosomal defects, stress, weight loss, excessive exercise, trauma, restrictive eating, and a family history of amenorrhea or early menopause. Pregnancy and breastfeeding cause secondary amenorrhea.	Weight gain, dietary changes, exercise restriction, birth control and other hormonal medications. If it is due to trauma or an eating disorder, cognitive behavioral therapy (CBT) is recommended. Surgery is only to correct a genetic or chromosomal defect, or to remove a pituitary tumor or uterine scar tissue.
	Sex, frequent douching, or using unclean sex toys.	Antibiotic tablets, gels, or creams put into the vagina, and abstinence until it clears up (even if your partner is a woman). Use mild soap or just water to wash, and if you use an IUD and BV recurs, try another form of birth control. Clean your vibrator more frequently and thoroughly.

Condition	What is it?	Symptoms	
Dysmenorrhea	A painful period with recurrent aching in the lower abdomen, back, or thighs before or at the start of your period. It can indicate another underlying condition that may impact your fertility.	Abdominal cramps, fatigue, nausea and vomiting, and diarrhea.	
Endometriosis	Referred to as the "missed disease," endo happens when endometrial cells proliferate outside of the uterus (usually in the pelvis), causing scar tissue, altered function of the fallopian tubes, and reduced egg reserves. Between one-third and one-half of women with endo have difficulty conceiving.	Painful menstrual cramps that originate in the abdomen or the lower back; painful sex, urination, and bowel movements; abnormal, heavy cycles with breakthrough bleeding; pelvic pain around your period; fatigue, diarrhea, nausea, constipation, and bloating.	

Causes	Treatment
Primary dysmenorrhea is caused by prostaglandins that cause the uterus's muscles and blood vessels to contract. Secondary dysmenorrhea is caused by endometriosis, pelvic inflammatory disease (PID), adenomyosis, fibroids, problems with the uterus and fallopian tubes, Crohn's disease, and urinary disorders.	Treating the underlying condition causing secondary dysmenorrhea clears it. Mild primary dysmenorrhea is treated with ibuprofen; oral contraceptives (if you aren't TTC); a heating pad; rest; avoiding smoking, caffeine, and alcohol; and trying yoga, massage, acupuncture or acupressure, mindfulness, and meditation.
No one knows for sure. Risk factors include having never given birth, low body mass index (BMI), early menarche, cycles less than twenty-seven days, and heavy periods longer than seven days, and hereditary factors.	NSAIDs and birth control can eliminate symptoms, and laparoscopy and keyhole surgery are used to remove out-of-place cells. If you are struggling to conceive, treatments start with ovarian stimulation medications and progress to IVF.

Condition	What is it?	Symptoms	
Polycystic ovary syndrome (PCOS)	Endocrine disorder that causes infrequent or longer than normal periods and amenorrhea. Polycystic refers to the small collections of fluid-filled follicles that form on the ovaries, preventing them from releasing eggs.	Unwanted hair growth, cystic acne, infrequent or missing periods, and polycystic ovaries are the diagnostic hallmarks. Others include heavy periods, weight gain in the abdomen, and pelvic pain. Symptoms are more severe in obese patients.	
Uterine fibroids (aka leiomyomas, or myomas)	Noncancerous growths, from tiny specks to watermelon-size masses that enlarge the uterus and fill the abdominal cavity. Fibroids are present in 10 percent of infertile women and can change the shape of the cervix and uterus or block the fallopian tubes, preventing sperm from reaching the egg.	Can be asymptomatic or cause heavy or long periods, pelvic pain, difficult or frequent urination, constipation, backache, leg pain, and a distended abdomen.	

Causes	Treatment
The exact cause is unknown, and it presents with varying symptoms. Like endo, it is hereditary.	Losing 5 to 10 percent of your body weight if you are overweight can reduce or eliminate symptoms, as can birth control. If you can't get pregnant, metformin or a fertility drug like Clomid, Femara, or injectable gonadotropins may be prescribed.
We don't know, though progesterone and estrogen appear to trigger their growth. They affect twenty-six million women between fifteen and fifty, and Black women are two to three times more likely to have them than white women.	Options range from expectant management (the wait-and-see method) to medications like anti-progestins, selective receptor modulators, IUDs containing progesterone, and gonadotropin-releasing hormone agonists (GnRH) removal procedures like a myomectomy, uterine artery embolization (UAE), and fibroid or endometrial ablation.

OTHER WAYS VAGINAL HEALTH
AFFECTS FERTILITY

Like the gut, the vagina is home to its own microbiome. A micro-biome is a set of microorganisms including bacteria and fungi that maintain a particular body part's equilibrium. Although there are more than two hundred different bacterial species that hang out in the vagina, the primary type is *Lactobacilli*, a form of bacteria whose acid inhibits the growth of bad bacteria. When *Lactobacilli* are in abundance it indicates the vagina is well-balanced. When the vagina is not dominated by *Lactobacilli*, vaginal dysbiosis, or imbalance, can cause problems like recurrent bacterial vaginosis or make you more susceptible to an STI or pelvic inflammatory disease. The vagina's pH changes over time based on hormonal fluctuations, pregnancy, menopause, sex, birth control methods, smoking, stress, and use of medications and supplements. One assessment of women from Asian, Black, Caucasian, and Hispanic ethnicities found that not only was the vaginal pH of women in these groups very different, but so too were the compositions of the vaginal bacteria communities, so it's hard to settle on one baseline that is ideal for everyone.

When it comes to fertility, research suggests that chromosomally normal miscarriages may sometimes be due to a lack of *Lactobacilli* causing mucosal barrier disruption, decreasing the vagina's defense mechanisms against pathogens. The ability of *Lactobacilli* to prevent infection in the vagina without inflammation is why we think it helps maximize fertility and promotes successful pregnancy outcomes. Around 40 percent of IVF patients have abnormal vaginal microbi-omes, and those with high levels of *Lactobacillus* were most likely to have success during IVF. *Lactobacilli* is a bacterium that occurs naturally in your body, and supplementing with it will not cause side effects. Best case, it may help reboot the vaginal flora. For menopausal women, vitamin D is shown to help vaginal health by improving the superficial epithelial cells and overall pH and decreasing dryness, and scientists assume some of the same benefits may translate in other age groups.

Dyspareunia, or painful sex, can happen to women during different parts of their reproductive life. It physically hurts and can cause negative emotional effects related to intercourse, so it should not be ignored. One reason it happens is a lack of vaginal lubrication thanks to hormonal fluctuations, which can be resolved with lubricant or more foreplay. Other times it's caused by involuntary spasms in the vaginal muscles, a condition also known as vaginismus. Vaginal and cervical infections, endometriosis, PID, and vulvodynia (chronic pain in the external sexual organs) can cause it too. And when you hit menopause, the vaginal lining can become less moist, which causes pain as well.

Before you pull out vaginal health products, douching does not restore your vaginal pH or microbiome, and you should only use soap and water on your vulva, no cleaning products need to go into your vagina. Ever. While it has an eons-long reputation as a home remedy for yeast infections and is delicious, putting a clove of garlic into your vagina will not cure anything. If you'd like to bathe in baking soda instead, it has proven antifungal qualities that kill the cells that cause yeast infections. The combo of Greek yogurt (no-sugar varietals only) and honey applied vaginally works more effectively than local antifungal agents to cure vulvovaginal candidiasis (a yeast infection in the vagina or vulva). Uncomplicated vulvovaginal candidiasis, which is 90 percent of cases, is handled with oral and topical treatments. Wearing cotton underwear is another way to keep your vagina healthy and works without the need to insert any foreign objects, foods, or other substances.

Menstrual Cycle Wrap-Up

- Use a cycle-tracking app or take notes to build a baseline of your cycle (and read the privacy policy before committing). Note characteristics like volume, color, regularity, and duration.

- Physical activity at varying intensity levels suited to each cycle phase helps manage many PMS symptoms and helps treat underlying conditions.

- Eat a diet packed with whole foods, leafy greens, olive oil, and whole grains.

- Improve sleep hygiene, especially around your period.

- BONUS: No clinical study proves that seed-cycling works, but there is no harm in trying it, and many PCOS sufferers swear by it. The basic version: during the follicular phase, consume one to two tablespoons of ground flax and pumpkin seeds daily to boost estrogen levels; then during the luteal phase, eat one to two tablespoons of ground sunflower and sesame seeds to promote progesterone production.

Chapter 2

EGGS

The amazing egg—
and what we can (and cannot) do to improve them

Early theories around the perpetuation of our species centered mostly around—surprise, surprise—male genitalia. Ancient Egyptians proposed that the sun god Ra masturbated or self-fellated the universe into being. The seed-and-field analogy popularized in the Talmud and Bible posited the man planted the seed and it was the woman's job to nurture it, a hot take that persists as women are still often treated as incubators. Other cultures believed that growing a baby required repeated infusions of semen throughout a pregnancy. Later, an epic debate raged in the seventeenth and eighteenth centuries between the spermists and the ovists who believed that their favored sex cell held a tiny fully formed human within, a concept called preformation. It wasn't until 1827 that the preformationists were silenced when the first undisputed observation of the human ovum was made by Karl Ernst von Baer, the father of embryology. He established that all mammals, including humans, develop from eggs.

The scarcity of eggs relative to sperm is one reason it is always in the spotlight when it comes to fertility. And while living in a reality that orbits less around testicles is refreshing, the pressure and responsibility for women to have perfect eggs is not. It's all about the egg, the egg is everything, the egg is all that matters. Until humans can reproduce without sperm, the egg is only one half of the equation. It is this humble author's belief that refreshment aside, we have gone a bit too far in the opposite direction.

With that said, the human egg is delicate, and the supply is finite. Women are born with all the eggs they will ever have, unlike men, who regenerate sperm constantly. Eggs that are genetically damaged cannot be repaired, and yes, age has the single biggest effect on an egg's quality. The reason: most problems with eggs are the result of errors during cell division, which happen more frequently as women age simply because the body becomes less efficient at it. These errors are the primary cause of chromosomal abnormalities. Chromosomally abnormal eggs cause delays in conception, miscarriages, genetically abnormal pregnancies, and failed IVF cycles. Other common causes of egg-related issues are conditions like PCOS and endometriosis, high insulin levels, and exposure to endocrine-disrupting chemicals like BPAs and phthalates.

Fertility starts to decline for women between ages twenty-five and thirty, then more significantly at thirty-two. There are nuances based upon lifestyle and overall health, but thirty-seven (not thirty-five!) is the age fertility truly drops for women, and the majority who try to conceive before that time will be pregnant within a year. The study that declared a woman's fertility withered away at age thirty-five was modeled using a data set gathered in rural France between 1670 and 1830. Since the time of the French Revolution, a few things—diet, lifestyle, chemical exposures, activity levels, norms around work, and life spans among them—have changed. The data was not representative of different ethnic or cultural groups, nor did it include women living in urban environments. Worth mentioning: egg-related (and all other) fertility research even now is not without flaws. The data we have is derived almost exclusively from IVF cycles, as infertility gets far more funding than natural conception. Although it seems like what works for IVF should work for natural conception, we don't know for sure because the studies have not been performed.

If you're undergoing fertility treatments and need a boost, some medications can increase the number of mature follicles and treat other conditions too. But there is no pill that will universally or exponentially improve your egg quality, and some come with unintended side effects. We'll cover supplements in the next section, but DHEA (dehydroepiandrosterone) is a great example of why chugging pills marketed to improve fertility without a clinician's guidance is not a good idea. DHEA is a popular fertility supplement, suggested by some clinics in the months before an egg retrieval to improve diminished ovarian reserve (DOR). Many women assume it is always fine to take, but it is only appropriate if your testosterone levels are low, and only if you have DOR. The dose is specifically based on testosterone levels, as taking too much for too long can interfere with egg development and cause side effects associated with high testosterone levels like oily skin, acne, and unwanted hair growth. Also worth mentioning: the United States is the only country where DHEA is available over the counter. In Europe, the United Kingdom, Australia, and Canada, for example, it requires a prescription.

Consider nurturing the healthiest eggs possible a by-product of working on your overall health in the three months before you try to conceive. And know that no matter how many supplements you take, salmon filets you eat, or other lifestyle hacks you try, there is no guarantee of a healthy pregnancy, baby, or fix to an aging egg supply regardless of how disciplined you are. With that, let's dig into egg basics: how they work, what goes wrong and why, what you can control about egg quality and development, and what you cannot.

> *My aging eggs were the most likely culprit behind our failed preg-*
> *nancies. I was over thirty-five when our fertility journey began, and*
> *my healthy and active life was no match for my body's decreasing*
> *ability to accurately perform cell division. I wish I'd been given the*
> *information below (versus the well meaning but vague diagnosis of*
> *"bad luck"). The majority of the time, miscarriage is due to chro-*
> *mosomal abnormalities, not stress or a fall or anything else you did.*

EGG FAQS

What is an egg?

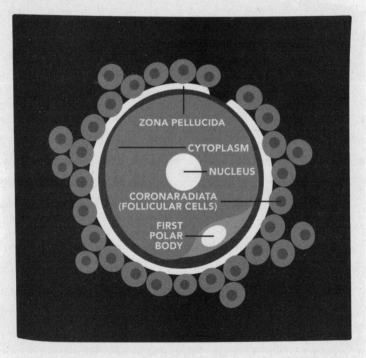

Eggs are biological marvels. Small to our eyes, a mere .1 millimeter in size, the egg is mighty. Compared to other cells in the body it is giant and holds half of everything required to begin human development. Yes, you're reading that correctly—an egg is a single cell, more specifically a sex cell known as a gamete. A potential, immature egg is called an oocyte. The corona radiata is the innermost layer of cumulus cells that forms a sunburst appearance with the maturing oocyte. Once the oocyte matures, those connections largely disappear. The zona pellucida is an acellular structure that surrounds the oocyte and serves as the species-specific barrier to fertilization. Going deeper you reach the cytoplasm, which is a gel-like substance that holds the cell's internal structures, or organelles like the powerful mitochondria. Then at the center is the nucleus that, just like sperm, holds the genetic material essential to create human life.

How many eggs do women have?

A human fetus forms approximately seven million oocytes in the womb. Women are born with around one million oocytes—all the potential eggs they will ever have—and lose around one thousand per month after puberty. Just four hundred to five hundred mature eggs are ovulated during a woman's life. At thirty-five, only around 6 percent of oocytes are left, and by menopause there are around one thousand.

Where do eggs come from?

An egg's journey begins before birth in the ovaries, where it lies dormant in a primordial follicle until menarche. At the start of each menstrual cycle, between ten and twenty primary follicles begin their growth. By day nine, only one healthy follicle remains; the rest are reabsorbed into the body. At ovulation, the wall of the follicle ruptures and the now mature egg is released into the fallopian tubes for fertilization.

What happens to an egg after it is ovulated?

Eggs only hang out for twelve to twenty-four hours in the fallopian tubes waiting for sperm. If no fertilization occurs, the egg is reabsorbed into the body. If it is fertilized, the egg and the sperm unite to make a single cell, known as a zygote. The zygote must then survive the journey to the uterus while dividing rapidly. When it becomes a blastocyst five to six days after fertilization, it will clock in at two hundred to three hundred cells before implanting into the uterine lining. If it does, a pregnancy begins. If it doesn't, the body reabsorbs the cells.

I haven't thought about cell division since biology class. How does that work again?

There are two types of cell division pertinent to this conversation: meiosis and mitosis. Meiosis is the process that creates eggs and sperm cells, or gametes. Each gamete holds twenty-three chromosomes, and when joined together, the combination holds forty-six (two of each) and the genetic basis for a future human. Mitosis is the process required to create every other cell in the human body. It works by replicating that combined parent cell into two brand-new identical cells.

So how does cell division impact fertility?

Errors in cell division, especially meiotic errors in eggs, are the primary cause of miscarriage, birth defects, genetically abnormal pregnancies, and other fertility issues like implantation failure. The quality of the egg and sperm cells that form the zygote (fertilized egg) are the first way things can go wrong, although meiotic errors are far more common in eggs than sperm, accounting for around 95 percent. That initial set of combined chromosomes is the template for the roughly two trillion cells that comprise a baby. After the first parent cell is created, it must then be replicated perfectly during mitosis over and over and over to result in a healthy baby.

Why do errors in meiosis happen?

An oocyte starts out with two copies of every chromosome. Before it can be fertilized, it must drop the extra copies during the first phase of meiosis. To do this, the cell's spindle apparatus pulls one copy of each chromosome to opposite sides of the spindle's pole. If the spindle pole is unstable or the cohesions between chromosomes are weakened (both scenarios happen more with age), chromosomes can be misarranged, resulting in too few or too many chromosomes in the mature egg. When an egg has one or more extra or missing chromosomes, it causes a condition called aneuploidy. The presence of an extra chromosome is called a trisomy, and a missing chromosome is called a monosomy. Aneuploid eggs that become fertilized usually end in an early miscarriage. If it does survive, it causes stillbirth or chromosomal conditions like Down syndrome.

How common is aneuploidy?

For women in their early thirties, between 10 and 25 percent of eggs are aneuploid. The number jumps to between 50 and 80 percent in women over forty, which is why there are more genetically abnormal pregnancies and miscarriages at and after that age. While meiotic errors are a cause of aneuploidy, they aren't the only ones. The mitochondria are the cell's powerhouse, and vital for proper egg and embryo development. As women age, their mitochondrial DNA (mtDNA) develops variations that alter its ability to fuel cells. This mutated mtDNA is then passed on to the embryo, which often cannot implant into the uterus as a result.

Can errors happen during mitosis too?

Yes, they can, and for the same reason—the body's ability to perform cell division becomes less efficient and more inaccurate as it ages. And accuracy is everything. When chromosomes do not halve equally during mitosis, it too causes aneuploidy and is responsible for cases of mosaicism. Mosaicism happens when there are two or more genetically different sets of cells in the body. When it happens early in human development, as many as 50 percent of cells can be abnormal, which often leads to miscarriage.

How do I optimize my body's ability to perform mitosis and meiosis?

One recent study showed that compared to other mammals, human eggs are deficient in a motor protein that helps to stabilize the spindle that separates chromosomes during cell division. Fixing this deficiency seems to increase the fidelity of the spindle and lead to more accurate chromosomal segregation. But it's all very experimental and, though promising, not available as a therapy today. Other than work happening in labs, there is no way to improve your body's ability to perform cell division. Going into conception with the healthiest lifestyle possible by following the advice in the next section is the best way to optimize your odds of success.

Why else is aging so rough on eggs?

Along with the arrival of crow's-feet, declining egg quantity is an inevitable part of aging. One hormone marker that indicates how many eggs are left (ovarian reserve) is anti-Mullerian hormone (AMH). It cannot tell you about their quality, but it does indicate how long until you may hit menopause and whether egg freezing or having a child should be on the horizon more immediately. It can be predictive of how successful IVF cycles will be too. Diminished ovarian reserves (DOR) do not mean you will never get pregnant naturally, as it only takes one high-quality egg to make a baby, nor is DOR associated with an increased risk of aneuploidy or lower live birth rates. However, when it comes to natural conception, DOR tells you how close you are to the end of your fertile years. If AMH is low and you'd like a baby or more than one child, the longer you wait, the less the odds are in your favor.

Are there other things that affect egg health?

Egg health is directly affected by exposure to certain medications and chemicals, lifestyle factors like smoking, pollution, and reproductive conditions like PCOS and endometriosis. There is a full list of must-avoids in chapter 9, but the most common are recreational drugs, tobacco, alcohol, toxic chemicals, plastics (BPA and phthalates especially), and radiation. Some health conditions like uncontrolled diabetes also have negative impacts. Chromosomal abnormalities that occur during pregnancy happen due to exposure to teratogens, or substances that cause or raise the risk of birth defects. Thyroid disorders can also cause miscarriages, and hypothyroidism (underactive thyroid) is linked to ovulatory dysfunction and premature ovarian failure. Thyroid-stimulating hormone (TSH) and thyroxine (T4) levels are part of a standard fertility workup, or you can do an at-home test if you're curious.

Can I test the quality of a single egg?

There is no test to evaluate the quality of an egg since it is just a single cell, and testing a single cell destroys it. Only embryos made during IVF—fertilized eggs that consist of multiple cells—can be tested to see if they are chromosomally normal. Those conceived naturally can only be analyzed during pregnancy with tests like noninvasive prenatal screenings (NIPT), chorionic villi sampling (CVS), and amniocentesis.

What about testing my overall egg supply?

There are a range of screenings, and typically a full hormone panel includes AMH, FSH, and estradiol since, in isolation, each marker provides limited information. Women with low AMH levels, for example, are sometimes told that they will not be able to get pregnant naturally. But low AMH alone is not a good predictor of overall fertility, nor are high levels a guarantee that it will be easy to conceive. FSH drives the growth of ovarian follicles. When it is out of the expected range for a woman's age, it can indicate natural conception or IVF treatments may be more difficult. High estradiol levels can also indicate a problem with ovarian reserves or egg quality. The most common test done in a doctor's office is a transvaginal ultrasound-led antral follicle count (AFC). It allows a physician to count the number of developing ovarian follicles and can reveal the presence of fibroids or endometrial tissue on the uterine lining.

How do I start with the healthiest possible egg?

Maturing healthy eggs comes down to living a healthier, fertility-friendly life since everything in your body is connected. So, unless you're undergoing assisted reproduction or know you have an underlying egg-related condition, start with lifestyle improvements. Pro tips and a full holistic program are in part two of this book. Yes, there is a slew of fertility products—from supplements to protocols and diets—that guarantee egg-related miracles like increasing ovarian reserves or the likelihood of conception no matter your age. But there is no magical cure for an aging or low-quality egg supply, just mitigation. If you want to try a few safe, side-effect-free options, CoQ10 is clinically proven to improve egg quality, so is getting more sleep to promote good melatonin production, eating a diet rich in antioxidants (and nixing processed foods), and avoiding endocrine-disrupting chemicals like BPAs and phthalates. Acupuncture can reduce stress and anxiety and may have other fertility benefits too.

When should I start optimizing my egg supply?

Instead of dropping your nightly glass of chardonnay a week before you TTC, commit to a healthier lifestyle over the long term. The cohort of follicles designated for growth is selected in the previous menstrual cycle, so for a full round of follicle production, egg optimization efforts should start three months or more before you try to conceive, just like sperm.

What should I know if I am thinking about freezing eggs to conceive later?

Preservation technologies have improved and are less expensive today, but conceiving with previously frozen eggs is not a certainty. See chapter 13 on fertility preservation for a full rundown on this topic, but a sobering retrospective study showed that the live birth rate for those who tried to use previously frozen eggs during IVF was just 39 percent. The retrieval process is a time-consuming and expensive surprise for many women too—and not without risk. To retrieve eggs from the ovaries requires ultrasound-guided insertion of an intimidatingly long needle through the vaginal wall, into the peritoneal cavity, and then puncturing each mature follicle in the hopes of recovering an egg. One round involves numerous visits to the doctor, eight to twelve days of hormone shots, a surgical procedure, and more than five thousand dollars, not including storage fees.

Eggs are amazing. Why do we need sperm anyway?

Virgin births are not a thing, and until science finds a way, the presence of sperm is a requirement for human reproduction. Parthenogenesis, or when a female gamete develops into an embryo without the male sex cell, is a form of asexual reproduction seen naturally in insects, a few species of sharks, crustaceans, and plants. It rarely works even when induced in mammals, and when it does, the offspring rarely develop normally.

Egg Wrap-Up

- Most problems in eggs happen due to errors during cell division, simply because the body is not as efficient at it as we age.

- There is no way to fix chromosomally abnormal eggs. To optimize their quality and get a sense of whether or not you are ovulating normally, follow the tips below starting three months before you plan to TTC.

- Start tracking your cycle (including ovulation), get more sleep (six to eight hours per night), follow a balanced diet based on whole foods, manage your insulin levels, engage in moderate activity (while stopping vigorous exercise, especially over long periods of time), hydrate, and take CoQ10 and a prenatal vitamin.

- Stop all smoking and drug use (including all forms of cannabis), moderate alcohol consumption to less than two drinks per day (or stop entirely), and avoid endocrine-disrupting chemicals, especially BPAs and phthalates, air pollution, and processed foods and drinks that contain trans fats and added sugars.

Chapter 3

SPERM

Sperm matters—and why sperm physicals could be the future of men's health

Saying the word sperm makes everyone squirm. Even its first researcher, Antonie van Leeuwenhoek, hesitated to share his discovery of strange "animalcules" in his semen with the wider scientific world in 1677, worried that his "observations may disgust or scandalize the learned." Van Leeuwenhoek ultimately did announce his conclusion: that sperm was a parasite that lived in semen à la tapeworm. This was the first of many entertaining but miscalibrated sperm-related conjectures. The infamous spermist sect of preformationist researchers posited sperm transported a tiny, preformed human to women for incubation. Others thought its presence stimulated a woman's body to manufacture babies. It took two hundred years and more advanced microscopes to confirm that genetic material from males and females are both required and combine to form a human. Today, our knowledge of these tiny cells that comprise half the genetic basis of human life has not kept up with the rest of medicine. We cannot even utter its name in mixed company, in ads, to loved ones, or really, anywhere else even though sperm is synonymous with male reproductive health.

Sperm is still seen as a primal biological yardstick for manliness and virility. Mentioning sperm health to friends, even in the context of an infertility journey, is taboo unless it's in the form of a joke. Because no one talks about it, sperm suffers from its share of misinformation, especially around its impact on fertility, pregnancy, and future children. One of the best examples: most people believe men can father children into their nineties since they produce sperm into old age. But men experience age-related fertility decline starting at thirty-five with a significant drop at forty, just like women. Between ages thirty and forty, men see a 52 percent decrease in their fertility rate due to degrading sperm. Every year of a man's life, sperm motility and morphology (normal size and shape) goes down, and DNA fragmentation (separation or breaking of DNA strands inside sperm) increases. In studies controlled for maternal age, first- and second-trimester pregnancy loss increases by 27 percent in fathers older than thirty-five and doubles in fifty-year-olds.

Sperm's concentration and count have also dropped precipitously—over 50 percent globally since the 1970s—for reasons unknown. Increased rates of obesity, lifestyle factors, and endocrine disruption are today's leading theories but we don't know for sure. Spermpocalypse, a scenario in which future men have little or no sperm, is unlikely, and for now overall sperm numbers appear to meet the basic requirements for human reproduction. So why care about this seemingly innocuous change? The quality of a man's semen correlates with his overall health. Poor quality has effects on women, families, and future children too. A father's age is the dominant factor in determining the number of new genetic mutations in a child. The risk of schizophrenia, Down syndrome, bipolar disorder, autism, childhood leukemia, other cancers, and genetic mutations increases with paternal age. So does the risk of a baby being born prematurely with lower Apgar scores (a test given at birth to indicate a baby's overall health) or having seizures or disabilities like congenital heart disease and cleft palate. Partners of men forty-five and older are at greater risk for gestational diabetes and preeclampsia during pregnancy. The theory is that just as a person's overall strength and fitness decline with age, so does sperm quality.

Let's dig into the reasons sperm quality may be falling. Exposure to endocrine-disrupting chemicals is at the top of the list, especially substances like phthalates and BPA that are commonly found in plastics, as well as microplastics. They are now found in human and fetal bloodstreams and are causing inflammation in nearly every organ system. Chemical exposures, combined with smoking, drug and alcohol use, and increasingly sedentary lifestyles make men's bodies a particularly inhospitable environment to manufacture and store sperm. And these changes are not just happening in humans. Dog semen quality has dropped, and genital anomalies where animals are born with intersex ambiguity have been observed in reptiles, and mammals like otters too.

The menstrual cycle is an excellent, easy-to-monitor indicator of a woman's overall health. Semen quality is a similar biomarker for men. And yet the challenge of managing men's health returns to the culture of toughing it out, which begins during childhood. The result is that only half of men consider a yearly physical or engage in any form of preventive care. Even when showing symptoms or nursing an injury, three in four prefer to wait before seeking medical attention. Since men would rather do anything else than go to a doctor's office, a yearly sperm physical taken from the comfort of home may be the simplest way to deliver more personalized, preventive healthcare. Tracking sperm statistics like morphology and motility along with DNA fragmentation, common in cases of male infertility, over time would build a more complete, true baseline of what's going on in men's bodies too, from individuals to the larger population. And in combination with environmental data, perhaps it would tell us more definitively why sperm is declining, how much of it truly can be tied to chemicals or lifestyle, or if it's something else entirely.

Beyond fertility, declining sperm parameters are a marker of other health trends, like low testosterone levels, tumors, cancer, diabetes, cryptorchidism (undescended testicles), and overall morbidity and mortality. Not great news, since men's life spans are five years shorter on average than women's and dropping at a faster pace. From consistency to the color, appearance, smell, and how sperm performs under the microscope, a semen sample can reveal a sexually transmitted disease and predict whether men will develop diabetes or heart disease or die early. Yet, our basic understanding of sperm—its genetic, cellular, biochemical, and molecular mechanisms—is surprisingly limited as research into male infertility is underfunded relative to other diseases. There is no medical specialty that manages men's reproductive health as gynecology does for women, either. Men have more long-term diseases to manage too, which creates huge emotional, social, and financial burdens on families, the healthcare system, and society. Men must become more engaged with their healthcare, get regular checkups, and upgrade their lifestyles. Men produce sperm nonstop, so with the right supplements and lifestyle modifications, some fertility issues are treatable.

Since male reproductive health isn't really covered in sex ed (or anywhere else) we'll start with sperm basics and how the male reproductive system functions.

SPERM FAQS

Okay, so what exactly *is* sperm?

Derived from the Greek word *sperma*, meaning "seed," they are male sex cells that carry half the genetic material necessary to create human life. Formed during a process called spermatogenesis, sperm regenerate constantly inside the testes and are ready for prime time after around seventy-four days.

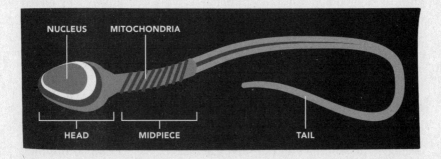

A single sperm measures just 0.0508 millimeter from end to end. The sperm head contains two compartments: the acrosome, a sac filled with enzymes that helps the sperm to penetrate the female egg, and the nucleus, which contains the all-important DNA. The neck holds energy-producing mitochondria for the sperm's torrid journey through the reproductive organs. And the tail is made of axial filaments powered by mitochondria that twist and propel the sperm to its goal—the egg.

Where do sperm come from?

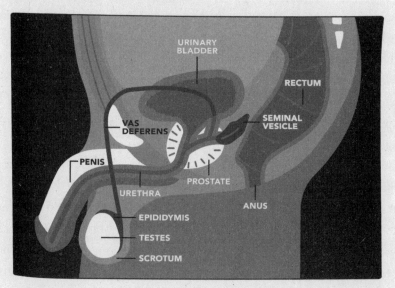

The male reproductive system's reason for existence is to manufacture, store, and transport sperm. Its component parts are the penis, testicles, duct system (epididymis and vas deferens), and accessory glands (seminal vesicles and prostate gland). Sperm start as germ cells in the testicles, housed in a system of tiny tubes called seminiferous tubules. Each testicle has seven hundred feet of this tubing, and it is there that they meet hormones like testosterone that convert them into sperm. After they divide and grow tiny tails and assume their tadpole-like appearance, spermatozoa take a five-week trip into the epididymis for storage, then move into the vas deferens to await their release. *Vas*

deferens is Latin for "carrying-away vessel," and that describes its purpose: to transfer sperm into the urethra where they combine with secretions from the accessory sex glands to form semen. Then, when it's time, this mixture is ejaculated.

Besides fertilizing an egg, what does sperm do?

Sperm dictates a baby's sex. Every egg contains an X female sex chromosome, but around half of sperm contain an X, and half a Y male sex chromosome, meaning there is almost always a 50 percent shot of having a boy or girl. If you're looking for hacks, there is only one that is highly speculative and still unproven. Y sperm are lighter and faster than X sperm, making them slightly more likely to reach an egg first. Since sperm can live in the reproductive organs for up to five days, some scientists believe having sex closer to ovulation benefits the Y sprinters, while doing it in the days before rewards the more durable X sperm (it's fun, but just reiterating that this is just a theory).

How fast do sperm travel?

A man named Horst Schultz famously claimed he shot a load eighteen feet and nine inches at a velocity of 42.7 miles per hour. Even though it was debunked, his legend inspired some men to train their pelvic floors (yes, men have pelvic floors too) to compete for the speed and distance ejaculation world record. We don't have an absolute answer to how fast sperm go when they get into the vagina, since sticking a radar gun or speed measurement device into the female reproductive tract is not really possible. Nor is performing an exact simulation in a petri dish, as much depends on the circumstances within the vagina. A study done on women going through surgical sterilization found that sperm made the trip to the egg in about five minutes when deposited directly into the vagina. Our best estimate from observational studies is that during unassisted conception, potent sperm move at a rate of five millimeters per minute (roughly 0.0001864 miles per hour), completing the centimeters-long obstacle course from the penis into the uterine canal in around ten minutes.

Why does it take so much sperm to get a woman pregnant?

The vagina's obstacle course and cervical mucus filters out all but around 2 percent of sperm. Just a few hundred of the around two hundred million sperm typically released in a single ejaculate make it through the uterus, which is enormous to the tiny sperm. Once they swim through the uterine cavity, they follow the sperm-attracting scent emitted by the egg through the fallopian tubes toward their final goal. Many sperm are sacrificed in service of their competitors, releasing enzymes that facilitate passage of (capacitated) sperm through the corona radiata to encounter the shell that surrounds the egg, called the zona pellucida. That collision causes sperm to blow their tops so they can penetrate through the zona and fertilize the egg.

How long does sperm live?

One myth that will not die is that women can get pregnant if there is sperm present on a toilet seat or toilet paper or in a pool or hot tub. While sperm can live up to five days in a woman's reproductive tract, they dry up quickly in the open air. The odds of enough sperm surviving hot chlorinated water (they hate heat), or inert sperm left on toilet paper making it to and through the vagina is pretty much zero. Having said that, "just the tip" can get a woman pregnant. Intrepid sperm deposited on the vulva, or in between the labia majora can still make its way through the vagina and past the cervix. Sperm that can no longer do their job are mostly broken down and reabsorbed into the body or released during a nocturnal emission, aka wet dream. When they are, reinforcements quickly step in to take their place.

What kills sperm?

While not convenient for cavemen or anyone in a profession that involves running while wearing a loincloth, the testicles sit in the scrotal sac outside of the body because sperm production is temperature-regulated. As temperature increases, sperm production decreases—heat is anathema to sperm. In insect models, a heat wave just five to seven degrees Celsius above the optimum temperature damages male—but not female—reproduction. Heat reduces sperm competitiveness and life span, and surviving sperm spawn offspring with shorter life spans. The aptly named substance spermicide, which terminates sperm entirely or just impedes their progress, is a well-known sperm killer. It is found in many lubricants and oils, so if you're trying to conceive, read the labels and try ramping up the foreplay, since the vagina provides its own lubrication. Another foe is air, which dries out seminal fluid and the sperm swimming in it. Exposure to laptops, phones in pockets, and heated seats in cars also grievously injure sperm. And the rumors are true: men who wear boxer shorts may have a 25 percent higher sperm concentration than those who wear tighter versions. Our best guess is that certain styles of underwear may increase gonadotrophin (hormones that stimulate activity in the gonads) secretion, resulting in higher serum FSH levels, but more research is needed.

WTF is semen?

If sperm are the swimmers, then seminal fluid is their pool, and the combination of the two found in ejaculate is semen. Seminal fluid is manufactured in the prostate gland, seminal vesicles, and urethral glands. It is composed of enzymes and fructose that fuels sperm. It's translucent with a white or gray tint and a viscous texture. The amount of semen in a single ejaculate is three milliliters, or a half teaspoon. Just 2 to 10 percent of semen is sperm. But it's a competitive field—there is an average of two hundred million sperm in one ejaculation. Semen is alkaline, and the vagina is acidic, so the alkalinity helps to create a more hospitable environment for those swimmers.

Wait, is pre-cum semen too?

The fluid known as pre-ejaculate is released before ejaculation and is not, in fact, semen. Produced in the Cowper's glands, this clear fluid's job is to lubricate the urethra of the penis, help semen exit, and counteract the acidity of residual urine in the urethra. Sperm are not released in pre-cum, but they can remain in the urethra if you ejaculated recently, which means though it's unlikely, a woman could become pregnant from pre-cum sans protection.

How does ejaculation work?

Contrary to how it's depicted in porn, ejaculation is a mechanical reflex controlled by the central nervous system that starts with mental or sensory sexual stimulation. Impulses from the brain and local nerves cause muscles in the shaft of the penis to relax and become engorged with blood, causing an erection. Muscle contractions then stimulate the emission and transport of sperm from the testes to the base of the penis. As sperm leave the epididymis, they are bathed in secretions from the seminal vesicles and prostate. At sexual excitement's peak, the muscles at the base of the penis contract, and the combination of seminal fluid and sperm is ejected out of the tip in several quick spurts.

Is ejaculation a male orgasm?

Not always, though the two usually happen together. Men can ejaculate without having an orgasm, and the reverse can happen too. Think of an orgasm as the feeling or sensation of pleasure and the ejaculation as the physical expulsion of sexual material. Though men can have "fake" orgasms, the real deal is associated with a faster heart rate, elevated oxytocin levels, and pelvic muscle contractions.

What are the most common problems with ejaculation?

Ejaculation problems fall into several categories. Delayed ejaculation takes a long time or doesn't happen at all and can be caused by diabetes or injuries and increasing age. With premature ejaculation release occurs too soon and can be caused by drugs or thyroid and prostate problems. Retrograde ejaculation is rarer but happens when semen flows backward into the bladder due to nerve or muscle damage to its neck, especially after prostate gland or bladder surgery. Ejaculation problems can be situational, acquired, or they can be lifelong issues that start at puberty.

How quickly does sperm regenerate after ejaculation?

Don't think of it as regeneration—it's more like a refill, with the resupply always standing by. The body makes millions of sperm each day, and each complete production cycle over several months results in more than eight billion sperm.

What if I don't ejaculate for a few weeks?

If you're worried that going a long time without a release will kill your sperm or somehow hurt your supply or ability to achieve an erection, don't be. Sperm with expired shelf lives are broken down and reabsorbed into the body or released during a wet dream. And with their demise, many sperm are waiting in the wings. That said, if you are TTC, sperm quality goes down during long periods of abstinence, especially after seven to ten days, so aim for a release at least every three to five days.

What happens if you masturbate too much?

The unsubstantiated ejaculation world record is sixteen times in twenty-four hours. The generally accepted limit is ten times in a single day, and too much ejaculation results in lower sperm count, which then makes it harder to conceive. There are other consequences too. Too much masturbation overworks and weakens the pelvic floor, resulting in pelvic pain, constipation, urgent or uncontrolled urination, and painful sex.

Does porn cause fertility problems?

Watching porn can be part of a healthy sex life, but six hours or more a week is considered a high consumption rate. Neuroscientists believe that porn addiction triggers the same neural processes as substance addiction, including the reward circuitry in our brains that controls dopamine levels. Watching porn also gets in your head and can lead to less sexual satisfaction with normal intercourse, increased anxiety, and depression, and can cause self-esteem issues for partners. Physically, excessive masturbation can cause erectile dysfunction and pelvic floor dysfunction.

Do I have to take Viagra if I have erectile dysfunction?

An alternative treatment that is gaining steam to treat erectile dysfunction is cognitive behavioral therapy (CBT), and the efficacy can be as good as pharmaceuticals like the little blue pill. The programs also include pelvic floor exercises, physiotherapy, and tools like mindfulness training, since stress and anxiety can trigger it.

Do recreational steroids hurt male fertility?

Steroid use causes what can be irreparable damage during men's peak reproductive years, and the problem is growing. Anabolic steroids are synthetic versions of testosterone; the word *anabolic* refers to its ability to build muscle. While historically they were utilized by elite athletes, today their primary use is to improve a man's appearance. Between 1 and 5 percent of the global population abuses anabolic steroids at some point in their lives. This estimate is loose because so few admit it. Most users are men in their twenties and thirties, many of whom suffer from low self-esteem. Thirty percent of users go on to be dependent on steroids, which leads to adverse physical and mental health outcomes and notable impacts on fertility. Side effects of steroid use include decreased sperm production, shrinking testicles, cancer, and aggression. After a few conversations with reproductive endocrinologists, you'll hear that steroid abusers frequently lie about their habit—to their partners, friends, and doctors—and even ignore the need to stop for nine to twelve months to let the effects dissipate for fear their appearance will change. Most do not know when they start using steroids that these side effects exist but are so hooked that they are later unable or unwilling to quit. If you are taking them for aesthetic reasons and thinking about or actively TTC, please stop. If you're taking them under a doctor's care, talk to your physician about your conception plans and timeline so you can find an alternative.

Anything else that can affect men's sperm and fertility?

Medications and preexisting health conditions. There are many examples, but we'll use type 2 diabetes to illustrate how the presence of chronic conditions wreak multiple layers of havoc. The onset of type 2 diabetes is usually during the reproductive years, and it reduces semen quality. The medication most commonly used to treat it causes a different set of issues. Metformin is the most prescribed diabetes drug in the world, with more than 120 million patients worldwide. And there is a link between fathers who took it three months before conception and boys born with major genital birth defects such as undescended testicles and urethral issues. Other medications including some antibiotics and several drugs that treat high blood pressure, ulcers, and rheumatoid arthritis can also hurt sperm production. If you're planning to conceive in the next year, make an appointment with your favorite medical provider and go in for that overdue physical. Do an audit of your medicine cabinet and talk to them about your conception plans. Even though sperm regenerates on a shorter time frame, it can take time to swap out medications and find a new one that works. And for a true baseline of your fertility, book a semen analysis online or through a clinic.

Is there hope for sperm?

Procedures like intracytoplasmic sperm injection (ICSI), gene therapies, tissue freezing and grafting, and sperm cell transplantation could help salvage male fertility. And induced pluripotent stem cells may completely turn human reproduction on its head. Pioneered by Nobel Prize–winning Japanese scientist Shinya Yamanaka, this approach takes mature somatic (nonsex-related) cells in the body and reprograms them into completely different cell types. Induced pluripotent stem cells made headlines when they were used to transform cells from a mouse tail into germ cells that resulted in a litter of mouse pups. We have yet to achieve the same result in humans, but the possibilities if we do—from reversing infertility to same-sex reproduction—are mind-bending.

Sperm Wrap-Up

- Sperm is a biomarker for a man's overall health, and a semen analysis is a simple way to build a baseline of male fertility.

- Sperm regenerates constantly and many parameters can be improved with lifestyle tweaks.

- To optimize sperm quality, follow the tips below at least three months before you plan to TTC.

- Get more sleep (six to eight hours per night), follow a Mediterranean diet (good fats, less sugar and processed foods), cut out all sugary beverages like soda, avoid endocrine-disrupting chemicals, engage in moderate exercise, and get outside (men who spend more than ninety minutes outdoors each week have 42 percent higher sperm concentration than those who do not!).

- Stop all smoking and drug use (including all forms of cannabis and steroids) and moderate alcohol consumption to less than two drinks per day.

- Steroid use ideally should stop nine to twelve months before you TTC.

- Avoid frequent saunas, hot tubs, hot batteries in laptops, phones in pockets, heated seats in cars— anything that regularly increases your scrotal temperature—along with cycling.

- BONUS: Fan of the cold plunge? Try scrotal cooling and freezer-friendly underwear as both have some evidence showing they improve sperm parameters.

By writing this book and talking about sperm I am already destined to be that mom. *And I'm not sorry. Men's health is a mess, and by the time they are old enough to read this I'd like sperm parameters to be on the way back up so I don't have to gift sperm freezing as a graduation present. Even if your body does not produce sperm, this issue affects all of us, and awareness is the only way that women will stop being the center of the fertility conversation. So please, if you have a male partner, son, brother, or anyone else who you care about who makes sperm, share this with them. If you are a man reading this in anticipation of a semen analysis, I get that all you can visualize are sticky magazines, and you're nervous about the possibility of an adverse result. But avoiding this simple, noninvasive test is a huge and expensive disservice to your partner, and you. Male factor infertility is much easier to test and treat, so if you're having trouble getting pregnant, go in for an assessment.*

Chapter 4

HORMONES

The tiny molecules that command your fertility

In the twilight of his life, the brilliant misfit scientist Charles-Édouard Brown-Séquard injected himself with a combination of fluids drawn from the testicles of guinea pigs and dogs. After a few weeks of this potent brew, Brown-Séquard pronounced himself rejuvenated, claiming he could lift heavier weights, sprint up stairs, and work late into the night. While his concoction did not work, as he died five years later in 1894, it was the first recorded endocrine therapy and motivated future research on sex hormones. A few decades later, through research in mice and pigs, Edgar Allen and future Nobel Prize winner Edward Doisy showed that ovarian follicles produce not only eggs but also the hormone estrogen. Progesterone, the other ovarian hormone, was discovered after Willard Allen and George Corner isolated a hormone they dubbed progestin in rabbits. At a special meeting of the Health Organization of the League of Nations in 1935, it was formally deemed "progesterone," and the rest is history.

Like so many words in the English language, *hormone* is derived from Greek, the word *hormao*, meaning "to excite." And that is exactly what hormones do: they are signaling molecules that flow through the body via the hormonal superhighway, aka the endocrine system, telling our cells and systems what they need to do to keep us alive while regulating physiology and behavior. They aren't just made in the ovaries and testicles. The brain makes them. The gut makes them. Bones make them. And the body's various glands make them too. Just like a key in a lock, each hormone docks onto a cell's receptors and delivers instructions, like reminding the body to eat (ghrelin), or moving sugar into the cells to be used as fuel (insulin), or preparing the body for sleep (melatonin), or growing bone, brain, and muscle (thyroxine).

Even though they are found everywhere and do many things, hormones are most associated with women and the notion of being hormonal. Ironically, progesterone and estrogen levels are at their lowest during a woman's period, and it is this lack of hormones that signals the uterus to contract and dispel its lining. Here's another shocker: men and women have a nearly identical set of hormones. From testosterone and estrogen to LH, each has a role to play for both sexes. These sensitive little molecules are very easy to throw off, and the resulting instability can ripple through your entire body. The chemicals that are increasingly found in our food, water, and environment, like BPAs and phthalates, can mimic or even block hormones from doing their jobs. Known as endocrine-disrupting chemicals (EDC), they are linked to conditions including cancer, endometriosis, early puberty, respiratory problems, and abnormalities in sex organs. Chapter 9 will help you identify and avoid these horrible substances whenever possible.

Let's break down exactly what "hormonal imbalance" means. A hormonal imbalance happens when there is too much or too little of one or more hormones. It's problematic because the endocrine system is large and interconnected, and when even a single hormone is out of whack, it can affect others too. The cause can be genetic, brought on by lifestyle factors, medications and health conditions, stress, trauma, or eating disorders, and hormone levels fluctuate as you age. The result of a hormone imbalance can be a standalone symptom like acne or irregular periods, or a medical condition like PCOS, diabetes, or infertility.

Hormone imbalances can cause weight gain, anxiety, and more rarely tumors and growths too. Some conditions like thyroid disease require medication, while others can be treated by changing your diet (eating whole foods with enough protein, fiber, and healthy fats while lowering sugar intake), exercising more, getting enough sleep, reducing stress, and quitting smoking. There are many, many supplements that claim to cure hormone imbalances, but very few have any clinical evidence. If you're dealing with multiple mystery symptoms and have not explored your hormones, skip the influencer-led miracle cures and try the above hacks. If nothing is working or you're having difficulty conceiving, book an appointment with your favorite medical provider, or consider at-home hormone testing if you're not ready to seek care.

AT-HOME HORMONE TESTING FAQ

Hormones and fertility are inextricably tied, and compared to other areas of medicine, our understanding of them is still new. The result is that the way we test and treat hormone issues is still evolving. Hormone testing is an important part of an infertility assessment and is done in a doctor's office or lab with specific protocols and timing. If you test with a doctor, when you do it depends upon whether you're doing a full workup or testing an individual hormone. In a medical setting your care will be personalized to your specific situation, and you will receive strict instructions and show up for testing on a certain cycle day. But now, at-home versions are available too. They are cheaper and require less blood but still require specific timing and are best for those who are just exploring their fertility for reasons we'll cover next.

How does at-home hormone testing work?

It's simple: order a test online, follow instructions, send back, and wait for your results. When choosing a company, screen for tests that are reviewed by a board-certified physician and allow you to opt into a telemedicine appointment with a fertility specialist to interpret results. Because hormone levels fluctuate so much, it's important to time the test appropriately to get an accurate result. Women must do their sticks on specific cycle days, and usually the company will ask questions about birth control or cycle regularity to inform that precise window. One advantage for women who hate needles (and really who doesn't?) is that at-home versions take less blood. The most common collection method is a dried blood spot, which involves pricking your finger with a lancet, then squeezing a few drops of blood onto a card to mail back for analysis. Some more extensive at-home tests refer out to labs where you'll do a normal draw in person with a phlebotomist or nurse. Results are generally back in seven to ten days.

Can I take my at-home hormone test to my doctor?

Most doctors do not have a clue what to do with the results of at-home tests, or they will look and then rerun them using their specific protocol. The accuracy of at-home tests can vary in quality depending on the maker of the test, the environment in which the test was taken (e,g., did the box get hot or take too long to get to the test maker), and whether it was done on the correct cycle day. Taking a test on the wrong day can result in inaccurate data. So, while it's a great tool and useful in helping you understand if you should seek medical care, it doesn't integrate well into the bureaucratic world of healthcare. At-home tests do not test every single hormone or marker that a full workup in a medical office would, nor does it involve a physical exam, so they cannot diagnose every issue on their own. These tests are only appropriate for women between twenty-one and forty-five, as they are designed for the years when hormone levels are more stable—after menarche and before the onset of menopause. Clinic-based tests are still the gold standard because the reference lab instrument and hormone assay kit are that particular physician's therapeutic decision-making tool set. The same assays on different machines can provide slightly different results.

How often should I hormone test?

Companies market AMH testing to women every six months just to "keep an eye on things." Since they're available to anyone who wants them and typically cost under $200, what's the harm minus the expense, right? For one, it turns out that hormone levels fluctuate a lot day-to-day, cycle-to-cycle, and pending what cycle day the test is performed. Even AMH, which was thought to have minimal variation versus other markers of ovarian reserve like FSH, varies up to 20 percent throughout the menstrual cycle. If you talk to most reproductive endocrinologists, the ob-gyns who specialize in fertility, they will tell you that a frequent testing cadence is not useful for most people with one exception. Hormone imbalances can be sneaky, and when new symptoms creep into your life, they can indicate there is an underlying condition in play. Symptoms to watch include new cystic acne, weight changes, gastrointestinal issues, excessive hair growth or loss, vaginal dryness, irregular or a full halt to periods, and breakthrough bleeding. All these symptoms indicate one or several hormone levels are too low or too high. If you feel like something is off, ordering a test or doing several over time is an option if you're not ready to see a doctor.

Is at-home hormone testing a thing for men?

Though they're advertised primarily to women, men can do basic hormone panels from home too. Sperm production and quality are dependent upon hormones being in balance, and in most cases, parameters can be improved given time and effort and knowing what's going on. Also, bonus: some male hormone screenings are done via saliva, not blood, so needle haters have no excuse. Male hormone tests generally focus on four markers: free testosterone (the biologically active form), cortisol (the stress hormone), estradiol (the main type of estrogen), and dehydroepiandrosterone (DHEA—the precursor to the other sex hormones). Men's fertility dips in their forties as they enter andropause, the male equivalent of menopause. It is caused by falling levels of testosterone, which declines naturally as men age. Most men produce sperm for the rest of their lives regardless of entering this life phase (though as we know, the quality declines over time), whereas menopause in women signals that the egg bank is empty and the baby-making years are over. Timing matters when it comes to hormone testing for men too, as testosterone levels swing every fifteen to twenty minutes and have daily, seasonal, and annual rhythms, so follow the instructions closely.

Okay, okay. So, should I try at-home hormone testing or not?

The best reasons to take these tests are curiosity and cost. Doing the same hormone panel in a doctor's office costs upward of $1,000 and is not covered if it's not diagnostic. Doctors aren't into doing tests just because you're curious; there must be a medical reason to order one and charge insurance. If you are looking for a baseline, general idea of your overall fertility, at-home tests are a great way to achieve that at a low cost. If you're looking for information beyond that or navigating infertility, it's best to book an appointment with your doctor. And if you are a data-driven person, just remember that more isn't always better and testing every month is unlikely to be helpful since hormone levels naturally fluctuate.

Female Hormone Cheat Sheet

Wondering what all these random hormones do in your body? Here is a quick guide to make sense of your test results, or to just nerd out on their functions. It's organized by hormone, and those that are mostly commonly tested on at-home and in-clinic panels are listed. As with eggs and sperm, the best way to improve your hormone levels is committing to a healthier lifestyle, though there are specific ways to handle diagnosed issues.

Hormone	What is it, and what does it tell you?	What can you do to improve it?
Anti-Müllerian hormone (AMH)	AMH levels do *not* reveal the ability to get pregnant naturally, just how much time is left before menopause. It is a measure of ovarian reserves, or the number of eggs left in your ovaries. High levels mean more follicles and eggs ready to ovulate, while low levels mean fewer. High AMH can indicate PCOS too. AMH is a good way to predict egg freezing and IVF outcomes.	Medications like clomiphene citrate, gonadotropins, and metformin that stimulate follicles and improve the likelihood of ovulation. Improving lifestyle factors—especially eating a healthy diet—helps too.

Hormone	What is it, and what does it tell you?	What can you do to improve it?
Estradiol (E2)	A form of estrogen that helps maintain the egg supply, stimulates egg and endometrial maturation, and levels up cervical fluid to be its most fertile around ovulation. High E2 levels can suppress FSH, which is why they are often tested together.	Eat foods like flax and sesame seeds and soybeans, which contain high levels of phytoestrogens; try supplements DHEA, vitamins D and B, and boron, or black cohosh and evening primrose oil. Talk to your provider before taking supplements, as there are interactions between evening primrose oil and several medications including antidepressants, and black cohosh can impact liver function and cancer drugs.

Hormone	What is it, and what does it tell you?	What can you do to improve it?
Follicle-stimulating hormone (FSH)	Grows the follicles that house eggs and prepares eggs for ovulation. It also stimulates the production of estrogen and progesterone necessary to maintain the menstrual cycle. High FSH levels can indicate ovarian reserves are decreasing.	Eat foods rich in omega-3 fatty acids like avocados, kidney beans, nuts, oily fish, and dark green leafy vegetables like broccoli, cabbage, kale, and spinach. Hormone-replacement therapy and surgery to remove tumors or cysts are reserved for serious cases.
Luteinizing hormone (LH)	Helps to regulate your cycle and ovulation. High LH levels can indicate ovarian failure and PCOS or genetic conditions. Low levels can point to a pituitary gland issue or are the result of malnourishment or disordered eating.	Improve lifestyle factors like diet, weight, and activity. If it's still low and you aren't ovulating, estrogen replacement, gonadotropin treatments (an injection of LH and FSH), and human chorionic gonadotropin (HCG) injections are medical options.

Hormone	What is it, and what does it tell you?	What can you do to improve it?
Progesterone	Known as the pregnancy hormone, it helps stabilize rich, thick uterine lining, triggers cervical fluid and waking temperature to change, boosts metabolism, and assists with brain function. Higher levels after ovulation indicate that an egg was released.	Reduce stress and body fat, do not overexercise, avoid EDCs, and eat a diet full of leafy greens, nuts, whole grains, and foods that contain zinc and vitamin B. Never use a progesterone supplement without a physician's guidance.
Prolactin (PRL)	It has more than three hundred functions in the body, including regulating metabolism and the immune system, but also indicates ovulatory issues. It stimulates milk production and pauses ovulation after pregnancy if you are exclusively breastfeeding. Too much prolactin in your blood when you are not pregnant causes hyperprolactinemia, which can bring about anovulation, and irregular or missed periods.	Improving prolactin levels is most applicable while breastfeeding, and done by eating oats and barley, which contain phytoestrogens and beta-glucan, or through medications.

Hormone	What is it, and what does it tell you?	What can you do to improve it?
Testosterone	Helps with the growth, maintenance, and repair of reproductive tissues and production of estrogen, and stimulates follicle growth, which is why it is important for egg freezing and IVF patients. High levels can indicate PCOS or congenital adrenal hyperplasia.	Lifting weights and resistance training, eating a well-balanced mix of healthy fats, protein, and carbs, and minimizing stress. Vitamin D3 supplementation boosts testosterone and so does getting it naturally via sunshine.
Thyroid-stimulating hormone (TSH)	Indicates how well your thyroid is functioning. One in eight women experiences imbalances like hyperthyroidism or hypothyroidism, which can be responsible for cycle-related issues, PCOS, and later pregnancy complications like miscarriage, preterm birth, and abnormal mental and thyroid function in babies.	Ensure your favorite health products and supplements do not contain biotin, which can cause a false reading as it's used to analyze your blood sample. Accutane, caloric restriction, glucosteroids, endocrine-disrupting chemicals, and milk thistle can drop TSH levels too.

Hormone	What is it, and what does it tell you?	What can you do to improve it?
Thyroxine (T4)	Helps the body control energy use and metabolism. If it's too high or too low, it can indicate hyperthyroidism, hypothyroidism, or hypopituitarism.	Steroids, birth control and other pills that contain hormones, thyroid medications, multivitamins that contain biotin, and some cancer drugs can affect T4 levels. Hypothyroidism is treated with a thyroid hormone pill; hyperthyroidism is treated with antithyroid medication, radioactive iodine, and sometimes surgery.

Male Hormone Cheat Sheet

Hormone	What is it, and what does it tell you?	What can you do to improve it?
Follicle-stimulating hormone (FSH)	Stimulates the testes to produce and transport mature sperm and can reveal sperm count. Low levels may mean insufficient sperm production while high levels can mean the testicles are not functioning properly. Levels don't generally fluctuate, so when FSH levels are off in combination with low sex drive or low sperm count, it causes infertility. When FSH is completely absent it can lead to azoospermia.	Reduce stress and avoid steroids and other hormonal drugs that contain testosterone. Disordered eating, a diet high in soy protein, and abusing alcohol also affect FSH levels. Hormonal replacement therapy is the first medical approach, but if it cannot be treated IUI and then IVF are indicated.
Luteinizing hormone (LH)	Stimulates the testes to make testosterone and indicates sperm production.	Improving diet, weight, and activity. Medications include gonadotropin treatments (an injection of LH and FSH) and HCG injections to stimulate the testes.

Hormone	What is it, and what does it tell you?	What can you do to improve it?
Testosterone	Affects libido and sperm health and production. Testosterone levels drop by an average of 1 percent every year after age forty. Low levels (hypogonadism) can cause low sex drive, erectile dysfunction, depression, and sometimes but not always decrease sperm production. High levels of testosterone (hypergonadism) can indicate steroid use, tumors, infection, genetic abnormalities, autoimmune disorders, injury, and cause low sperm count and infertility.	Lifting weights and resistance training, eating a well-balanced diet of whole foods, and reducing cortisol levels by diminishing stress. Supplements include vitamin D3 and ashwagandha, an Ayurvedic herb. Testosterone replacement therapy lowers sperm count as it impacts other hormones. Unless you're under a doctor's guidance (and please speak to them if you are before you TTC), stop taking anabolic steroids and any testosterone supplements.

Hormone Wrap-Up

- A hormonal imbalance happens when there is too much or too little of one or more hormones. When even a single hormone is out of whack, it can affect others too.

- The cause can be genetic, brought on by lifestyle factors, medications and health conditions, stress, trauma, or eating disorders, and hormone levels fluctuate as you age.

- A hormonal imbalance can have symptoms like acne or irregular periods, lead to a medical condition like PCOS or diabetes or infertility, and can cause weight gain and anxiety too.

- Easy ways to improve imbalances are eating whole foods featuring protein, fiber, and healthy fats while lowering sugar intake, exercising more, getting enough sleep, reducing stress, and quitting smoking.

- There are many supplements that claim to cure hormone imbalances, but very few have enough clinical evidence to support their use.

- At-home hormone testing is useful if you are curious about your fertility or you suspect something is off. But if you need to seek fertility care your doctor will re-run hormone panels on their own equipment.

Chapter 5

BIRTH CONTROL

Understanding different types of contraception and the effects (or not) on your fertility

The earliest written record of birth control was inked on Egyptian papyrus around 1550 BC. The authors noted that a combination of honey, lint, and acacia leaves, renowned for their spermicidal qualities, placed into the vagina prevented pregnancy. A pessary consisting of crocodile dung or exclusively breastfeeding for several years were other proposed solutions. In the book of Genesis, the pullout method is referenced when Judah's second son, Onan, refused to follow local customs and give his dead brother's wife a child. It didn't end well for Onan—God smote him down for his disobedience. But this episode inspired the phrase "spilling seed on the ground," or ejaculating without reproductive possibility, which in some religions is still considered a sin. In ancient China, coitus reservatus, or pulling out but not ejaculating, was considered superior as it was believed that spilling your seed caused a loss of yang, the essence of masculinity. If you could avoid ejaculating, vaginal sex was viewed as beneficial to men's health, as it allowed them to receive yin, or feminine energy, thus restoring balance in their bodies. Until inventions like barrier methods and hormonal birth control, coitus interruptus was the most effective way to ward off babies, as alternatives were as varied as inserting herbs into the vagina, drinking lead or mercury (which often resulted in death), and sporting weasel feet, the anus of a hare, or desiccated cat livers around the neck.

Our relationship with birth control through the ages was, like today, motivated by politics and religion, as it is more strongly associated with enabling sexual pleasure than preventing pregnancy. It wasn't until 1965 that the Supreme Court ruled in *Griswold v. Connecticut* that unmarried couples could possess and use contraceptives in the same ways that marrieds could. And now, there are more options than ever . . . for women anyway. Until hormonal male birth control is a thing, the perils of human reproduction and allowing it (or not) still fall to women. While exciting options are in the works, we are still a long way from a commercially available treatment that suppresses production of or blocks millions of sperm each day. Today's male birth control options are barrier methods (condoms), vasectomies, and the pullout method (bad idea, friends). It's a shame because there is a very willing market for a medical option. Over half of men say that if birth control sans side effects were available, they would happily take it. Women would also like birth control sans side effects and are in favor of male birth control, with 98 percent saying that they would trust their committed partner to use it.

It's not like science hasn't given it a shot. In the 1950s, a drug called WIN-18446 stopped sperm production in mice. When it was administered to humans, in this case inmates of an Oregon prison, a problem arose. While it completely blocked an enzyme called ALDH that helps produce sperm, it also froze another type of ALDH, which metabolizes alcohol. One test subject made an unfortunately timed choice to consume whiskey while on this treatment and nearly died of alcohol poisoning.

In the 1970s, a combination of synthetic testosterone and progesterone was shown to be effective in reducing sperm counts but came with too many side effects—side effects that are, ironically, like those reported with women's birth control pills. There are birth control injections, transdermal gels, and even a male IUD in the works, but none are effective enough, nor are they as reversible, affordable, or available as the pill. But there is hope: scientists are tinkering with different hormone combinations and attempting reversible reprogramming of sperm to be worse swimmers. Another promising treatment is a gel rubbed on the shoulders each day that cuts sperm count down to almost zero. Whether men adhere long-term to this daily birth control massage remains to be seen. Triptonide, a natural compound purified from a Chinese herb called Tripterygium wilfordii Hook F, is another nonhormonal possibility. It has been tested in mice and monkeys and causes the production of deformed sperm with minimal or no motility that cannot move enough to reach an egg. Four to six weeks after this oral medication is stopped, full sperm movement is restored, and no negative side effects have been recorded. But replicating the result of an animal trial in humans isn't always straightforward, and as we learned with WIN-18446, there can be unintended consequences to biological tinkering.

Hormonal birth control for women has changed a lot since it was invented, especially the pill—from formulation to ingredients and their levels. But myths about its side effects, from causing cancer, sterility, weight gain, acne, and other serious health issues are still going strong. Thirty-seven percent of women under twenty-five, for example, believe long-acting birth control (LARCs), a category that includes IUDs and injections, cause infertility. Only two-thirds of the same group knew that LARCS were a contraception option for those without children. We know definitively that no form of birth control on the market today causes cancer or infertility, but its more subtle side effects are still an open question. Efforts to link mood and emotional changes have so far been inconclusive or not supported by clinical research. The weight gain that women fear is temporary fluid retention, not fat. Early versions of the birth control pill were made with higher doses of estrogen, which could cause increased appetite, but today's have far lower levels. To prove any of this conclusively, a gold standard study that enrolls thousands of women who consent to be tracked over a year or more would need to be funded by independent researchers. That study design is unlikely to be implemented, since the placebo group would be susceptible to unwanted pregnancies.

About half of pregnancies are unintentional. 257 million women around the world want to avoid pregnancy but are not using safe, modern forms of contraception. 172 million women use nothing because they are afraid of infertility or hemorrhage, are opposed to contraception for religious reasons, are breastfeeding with no period and think they don't need it, and 24 percent just don't have sex. A lack of access and inability to pay for contraception are also major factors. Sixty percent of unintended pregnancies end in abortion, and 45 percent of abortions conducted worldwide are unsafe and lead to millions of hospitalizations. It's estimated that between 4 and 13 percent of maternal deaths are attributed to unsafe abortions. No matter where you sit on this issue, we should all agree that open, affordable access to birth control is necessary should we wish to see the abysmal trends in maternal mortality improve.

HORMONAL BIRTH CONTROL

Most unintended pregnancies that happen while on hormonal birth control are due to human error—not because it doesn't work. Human error manifests mostly as not taking medications on time as prescribed. Not all birth control methods are sexy either—some involve gels and goop and uncomfortable insertion, which can be a vibe killer. Most people don't know sperm can live for five days in the reproductive organs, which makes identifying the wrong fertile window (or thinking it's shorter than it is) another leading cause of accidental pregnancy.

Despite rumors to the contrary, all forms of birth control are reversible and have no long-lasting effects on your fertility. With natural birth control or barrier methods like condoms, there are no hormones involved, meaning that there is no delay back to normal fertility—you're good to go. With hormonal birth control, there is some timing to navigate, although most menstrual cycles and ovulation restart within three months if not immediately.

How does hormonal birth control work?

When used on time and correctly, hormonal birth control simulates aspects of pregnancy and changes cervical mucus quality to make it inhospitable to sperm. Hormonal birth control options break into two categories: short-acting hormone treatments and long-acting contraceptives (LARCs). The first is daily or monthly-use birth control options like pills, the patch, a shot, or a vaginal ring. Longer lasting (but still reversible) options include the increasingly popular IUD and implant and patch. Even if you've spent the majority of your adult life on one type of hormonal birth control, there are new tests that can assess whether they are the best option for you. Using saliva and blood samples, they test your genetics and hormones, combining the results to recommend the best type. They also predict which formulations will be most likely to suppress your period if that's a goal.

Some birth control options categorized as "user-controlled" like the pill, patch, and rings, can be purchased online. IUDs and implants require a trip to see a provider as they are not self-service. The shot falls somewhere in between, as some providers will write a prescription for the self-administered version. Telehealth-facilitated birth control is just as safe as going to see a provider in person, and it may even be safer, as undercover researchers found when they claimed to have a condition that would make hormonal birth control unsafe, 93 percent of the time a prescription was not given. In-person care achieves that standard 91 percent of the time. It is vital that, just as seeing a provider in real life, you are completely honest about your medical history and risk factors and any questions they ask so they can help you choose the right formulation.

The pill

What is it? Starting shortly after menarche, the pill can be prescribed to treat period symptoms and irregular cycles. It works by mimicking pregnancy, raising hormone levels that then suppress ovulation. No egg, no pregnancy. While the added hormones can help women as young as fourteen with intense period symptoms, it's worth noting that irregular ovulation, which is common in the first three years after menstruation starts, resolves with age. If you start combination pills (powered by progestin and estrogen) during the first five days of your cycle, you're protected the same day. If you start any other cycle day, it takes a week for the effects to fully kick in. Starting a regimen of progestin-only (POP or minipills) can happen on any cycle day and it takes forty-eight hours for them to become effective. It's a good idea to take the pill at the same time every day so it becomes a habit. With progestin-only versions it's necessary to take it during the same three-hour window every day for full protection.

Efficacy: With perfect adherence the pill is 99 percent effective. But most people miss pills or do not take them on the same schedule, so true efficacy is closer to 91 percent. Failure rates are greatest in women with a BMI over thirty-five.

Side effects: Many women state that getting on birth control makes them cry more easily, feel emotionless or disinterested in sex, or more anxious. These symptoms are worth paying attention to but not enough to make a depression diagnosis. Mood changes are a tough thing for researchers and pharmaceutical companies to study since only negative effects are reported. Mood is also affected by seasons and life changes, like a new sexual relationship and all the complexity that brings. Formulation differences can make a huge difference too. Some women who do poorly on estrogen versions do well when it's progestin only. In other words, we have a lot of anecdotal reports of mood changes with hormonal birth control, but no true clinical evidence since it's difficult to perform the appropriate studies. That does not mean your experience or your feelings are invalid. If you think the pill is causing negative changes to your mood, talk to your prescribing physician. Most encourage staying on it for three months to let things settle out. But if it is causing extreme side effects or you don't feel heard by that person, see someone else—and it may be time to try another formulation.

Time back to normal fertility: Some studies report long-term users of birth control have greater fertility; others conclude it's the same as those who have never taken it. But in general, there is only a transient delay—an average of around three cycles until full fertility is back and it's possible to get pregnant the cycle after you stop.

The patch

What is it? Usually placed on the butt, back, upper arm, or abdomen, the patch releases estrogen and progestin to stop ovulation and thickens cervical mucus to halt sperm. The hormones are absorbed through your skin, which means it must be placed and stuck on completely.

Efficacy: When used perfectly the patch is 99 percent effective. Because most people aren't perfect, and it's a physical sticker on the skin, it is closer to 91 percent effective. Reapplying patches that are no longer sticky, not sticking it on tightly enough, or forgetting to change it on time are the main problems. As with the pill, if your BMI is over thirty-five, there can be decreased efficacy.

Side effects: Most side effects happen in the first two to three months and are minimal. On the positive side, the patch generally makes periods lighter and more regular, or even nonexistent and can ease PMS symptoms like cramps. Negative side effects include headaches, nausea, sore breasts, spotting, and itchiness or other skin reactions around the spot where it's placed.

Time back to normal fertility: An average of four cycles after you stop sticking.

The shot

What is it? Powered by progestin, the birth control shot is an injection given every three months, usually by a nurse or doctor (though there are formulations you can self-administer at home), into the arm or your butt. The shot requires no daily management, just remembering to make (and keep) appointments or jab yourself on schedule four times per year.

Efficacy: The failure rate for women who get the shot on time is just 0.3 percent, making it one of the most effective birth control options available.

Side effects: It is known for irregular bleeding, somewhere between spotting and a period that can last for three months or more. Other side effects include nausea, nervousness and anxiety, migraines and headaches, fatigue, and dizziness, though they are rare. After a year, half of the people who take it have no periods. Because hormone levels are kept so low with the shot, there is a concern that it may cause thinning of the bones, a condition called osteoporosis. Studies on this topic are inconclusive, but you will probably run into this claim if you google. If you do experience bone loss, it rebounds to normal levels as soon as you stop the shot, so there are no long-term consequences.

Time back to normal fertility: While it is fully reversible, the shot has the longest timeline back to normal fertility, taking an average of five to eight cycles after stopping for most people to conceive.

The ring

What is it? The birth control ring, vaginal ring, or "the ring" is another solution that requires little upkeep and works for up to five weeks at a time. It releases a combination of estrogen and etonogestrel, a different form of progestin than is found in other combo pills, that stops ovulation and thickens cervical mucus. Follow the instructions of the manufacturer, but a good guideline is that rings need to live at room temperature, and any you are stockpiling for use after four months should be refrigerated.

Efficacy: Perfect use achieves a 99 percent effectiveness rating but due to human error, it's more like 91 percent. It's critical that the ring be put in on time every cycle and not left out of your vagina for too long, pending that formulation's instructions. If you're planning to use vaginal products, you can only use those that are water-based — no creams and gels, as they reduce the efficacy.

Side effects: Negative effects include headaches, nausea, sore breasts, spotting, and vaginal discharge. For those interested in period suppression, the ring typically eases heavy and irregular periods and symptoms like cramping. One rumored side effect is weight gain, but clinical studies do not support gain or loss.

Time back to normal fertility: Like the pill, the ring has a transient delay of around three months to normal fertility.

The hormonal intrauterine device (IUD)

What is it? This is one of today's most popular options and for good reason. It's easy, lasts for years, has few side effects, and is 99 percent effective in preventing pregnancy as it eliminates most opportunities for human error. There are multiple brands, all of which are formulated differently, and also copper IUDs which contain no hormones and are covered in the next section. Hormonal IUDs work by thickening cervical mucus and stopping ovulation. The insertion process starts with a speculum that goes into your vagina, and then a nurse or doctor uses a special tool to stabilize your cervix. Your practitioner will then insert the IUD into your uterus. The whole procedure takes around five minutes.

There can be cramping and pain when the IUD is placed, and some people get dizzy and a few faint, but discomfort generally lasts only a few minutes. It's still best to plan to take it easy after your appointment. You may notice a string one to two inches long coming out of your cervix. It's there for eventual removal, so do not treat your IUD like a tampon, as it is possible to pull it out or slip it out of place. How soon you can start having unprotected sex depends upon the manufacturer of your IUD, so use backup and check the official notes.

Efficacy: An IUD is 99 percent effective because there's little possibility of making a mistake or forgetting anything. All you need to do is track its expiration date and not pull it out.

Side effects: Cramping and spotting, especially in the first three to six months. Hormonal IUDs reduce PMS symptoms and make periods lighter (10 percent of women have no period). About one in twenty IUD users experience unexplained expulsion where it falls out. This is most common during the first three months and during your period. If it falls out its pregnancy-preventing powers are no longer in effect, so use backup birth control if that happens. It's important to get a displaced IUD fixed quickly, and you'll want to anyway as it can be uncomfortable.

Time back to normal fertility: Immediate—you can get pregnant the cycle after an IUD is removed. There is no negative effect or delay to conception. The only issue, which is present with all birth control options that treat period symptoms, is that you may not know about them, and symptoms can worsen over time.

The implant

What is it? Around the size of a matchstick, a birth control implant is inserted into your arm and, for the next five years, protects against pregnancy. This thin rod releases progestin, which thickens cervical mucus and stops ovulation. Right before it's inserted, your provider will numb the area with a shot, then use an inserter tool to gently slide the implant under your skin. It starts working immediately if you have it inserted during the first five days of your cycle, but otherwise you need to use a backup method for the first week. When you hit the five-year deadline or want to conceive, the removal process is the reverse of the way it was inserted. A numbing shot is given, then your provider will make a small cut and pull it out.

Efficacy: The implant is at the top of the efficacy pile—it prevents pregnancy 99 percent of the time. The reason it's so foolproof is that it just sits in your arm, quietly releasing hormones, and does not require any maintenance or daily diligence.

Side effects: Spotting is the most common negative side effect, especially in the first six to twelve months after its insertion, and it sometimes causes longer and heavier periods. But most users report that their periods get lighter or disappear entirely. Rare side effects include breast pain, headaches, nausea, water-weight gain, and ovarian cysts.

Time back to normal fertility: Just like the pill, you can get pregnant the cycle after it is removed.

The morning-after pill

What is it? Only intended to be used as emergency contraception, around one in nine women has used it, in some cases because they don't have health insurance and can't afford the pill. The main fertility misconception is that using it even once makes you infertile. Not true. The morning-after pill delivers a megadose of the very same hormones found in the pill to prevent the ovulation and fertilization of an egg and fertilized eggs from implanting into the uterus. It does this by thickening your cervical mucus so much that it stops sperm in their tracks, then makes the endometrium thinner and less embryo-friendly. Your period showing up is a sign that those hormones are no longer in your system and there are zero long-term effects or impacts on your fertility.

Efficacy: The morning-after pill is 89 percent effective when taken correctly and on time, and that timing changes based upon the formulation. The cutoff for emergency contraception options is no longer than 120 hours or five days after you had unprotected sex, but the closer you take it to the encounter, the better. And crucial note: it only protects against sex you've already had, not future sex, and you can get pregnant the day after taking it. If you plan to have sex again, use a barrier method. Some forms of the morning-after pill work less well if your BMI falls into the obese category, so speak to a provider to choose the one that is best for you.

Side effects: Though not universal, some women experience abdominal pain, nausea, irregular bleeding, breast tenderness, moodiness, headache, and fatigue.

Time back to normal fertility: Immediate, so always use a backup method if getting pregnant is not your goal.

BARRIER METHODS

Egyptian artwork and cave paintings in France revealed the invention of condoms fifteen thousand years ago. Giacomo Casanova (yes, he was a real person and renowned for womanizing) famously used assurance caps, the predecessor to modern condoms. Back then, they were used more for avoiding syphilis than contraception and the first versions were like gift wrapping a penis, as they were constructed of linen, soaked in a chemical solution, and tied on with a ribbon. Condoms went through a few iterations before today's versions emerged and were made of everything from lamb intestines, rubber (condoms earned that nickname for a reason!), and animal horn before manufacturers settled on latex.

Now they're made for her pleasure, his pleasure, studded, ribbed, scented, flavored, and coated with CBD. Their job, like all barrier methods, is to physically block sperm from progressing through the cervix. Other options include diaphragms, sponges, cervical caps, and spermicide, and the efficacy of each ranges between 70 and 88 percent, pending the additional use of spermicide. One bonus of barrier methods is that they all reduce (but do not eliminate) the risk of STDs, especially condoms when used correctly. And since none of them have lasting effects on the body, there is no impact on fertility—you can get pregnant immediately.

Condoms

What are they? Male condoms fit snugly over the penis and capture semen and pre-cum before they can go anywhere. Female condoms, while less common, are pouches made of polyurethane and inserted into the vagina.

Side effects: No official side effects, other than some physical discomfort and rare reactions to certain ingredients. Some men and women do not like the feeling of condoms, or the perceived reduced sensation during sex. But a bonus is that they can delay ejaculation, helping sex last longer.

Efficacy: Male condoms are around 82 percent effective, female condoms drop to around 79 percent.

Diaphragms

What are they? Diaphragms are shallow, reusable bowl-shaped cups worn inside the vagina and are usually used in combination with spermicide. They require a prescription and must be inserted before sex and worn at least six hours after vaginal sex for a maximum of twenty-four hours.

Side effects: Occasional physical discomfort while inserting or wearing, and increased risk of urinary tract infection (UTI). When left in your vagina for more than twenty-four hours, diaphragms can increase the risk of TSS.

Efficacy: Diaphragms work 88 percent of the time when used with spermicide.

Cervical caps

What are they? Like diaphragms, they are reusable (for up to one year when maintained properly), used in conjunction with spermicide, and made of rubber. They fit snugly against the cervix and look like a tiny sailor's cap, hence their name. Cervical caps can be worn for two days before coming out.

Side effects: Occasional physical discomfort inserting or wearing. Like diaphragms, if a cervical cap stays in the vagina for too long it can create an increased risk of TSS.

Efficacy: Cervical caps are 71 to 88 percent effective with typical use and spermicide. If you've given birth before, this is not the best option, as pregnancy and childbirth physically change your cervix.

Contraceptive sponges

What are they? Contraceptive sponges are small, round pieces of squishy medical-grade sponge (not the type you use to wash dishes) that contain spermicide. Like other barrier solutions, it is a physical impediment between your cervix and incoming sperm, used by itself or with additional spermicide. The sponge can be inserted up to twenty-four hours before you plan to have sex but must come out on the same timeline.

Side effects: Because the sponge can irritate your vagina, germs have an easier time hanging out and entering your body, so it can increase your risk of STDs and HIV. There is also some increased risk of TSS, and an ingredient that powers the sponge's spermicide can cause irritation.

Efficacy: Sponges are 73 to 86 percent effective when used as indicated and effectiveness rises based upon whether spermicide is used.

Spermicide and vaginal gels

What are they? Creams and gels put into the vagina before sex to slow sperm from reaching the egg or block the cervix. They work similarly, but spermicide comes in more form factors than vaginal gels, from creams, films, foams, and gels, to suppositories. Even though they are chemical compounds, neither are powered by hormones, which is good for anyone seeking to avoid those side effects.

Side effects: The chemicals in creams and spermicides can cause irritation, and some people have allergies to their ingredients. Spermicide can change the quality of cervical fluid too, making it more difficult to interpret if you are using a fertility-awareness method as your main form of birth control.

Efficacy: Spermicide is 79 percent effective when used alone.

COPPER IUD

What is it? The copper IUD lasts for up to twelve years and doesn't contain any hormones. Sperm hates copper enough that it's a very effective deterrent. Like a hormonal IUD, insertion takes around five minutes and is a lot like getting a Pap smear. Cramping and discomfort are common but generally only last for a few moments. You'll have a one- to two-inch string hanging out of your cervix for later removal, so don't pull on it.

Efficacy: The copper IUD is 99 percent effective because there is no maintenance, other than tracking its expiration date and leaving it alone.

Side effects: More intense cramping, heavier periods, and spotting, especially in the first three to six months. The first three months after insertion around one in twenty IUD users experience unexplained expulsion. If it does, use a form of backup birth control and get it fixed fast.

Time back to normal fertility: You can get pregnant immediately after a copper IUD is removed.

THE PULLOUT METHOD

What is it? Falling squarely into the "not a great idea unless you want to get pregnant" box, right as a man is on the cusp of ejaculation, he pulls out and finishes up outside the vagina. That's it. Because it relies so heavily on timing and discipline (especially his), this method is only okay if you are fine accidentally getting pregnant.

Efficacy: As many as one in four women (failure rates range from 22 to 27 percent but could be higher) who utilize the pullout method as their only form of birth control get pregnant each year.

Side effects: Falling whoopsie pregnant, making a mess (unless you're into it).

THE RHYTHM METHOD

What is it? Sometimes called natural family planning, the rhythm method relies on a woman's ability to correctly identify the fertile window and avoid sex or use barrier methods like condoms as backup during that time. Tracked using a calendar, the rhythm method is used if there are religious objections to other birth control, or for people who dislike or can't tolerate hormonal birth control. It relies on at least six months, preferably longer, of tracked cycle data, and an eleven-day-long period of abstinence or another form of backup birth control during fertile days to be effective. Because it's so reliant on an accurate fertile window, it's best to extend it a bit on either side since sperm can live in the reproductive tract for up to five days. If you do not have regular periods, it is hard to know your exact window unless you are diligently tracking every month or using an OPK.

An alternative that shares the same ethos is the standard days method, which for a twenty-eight-day cycle suggests days one through seven are not fertile, days eight through nineteen are fertile, and days twenty to twenty-eight are not fertile either. This only works if your cycles are regular and the duration of each is between twenty-six and thirty-two days. Pulling out is not a reliable backup method—try condoms or another barrier method.

Efficacy: It is effective around 76 percent of the time with no backup methods.

Side effect: Accidental pregnancy.

FERTILITY-AWARENESS METHOD (FAM)
OR SYMPTOTHERMAL METHOD

What is it? This one takes the rhythm method a step further, combining cycle tracking with two other pieces of data: basal body temperature and cervical mucus. FAM requires strict adherence to be effective, and the best results are achieved by using a combination of all three, which is called the symptothermal method. FAM is only recommended for those in monogamous relationships with the discipline to track all three data points every day.

The temperature method: Your basal body temperature (BBT) changes throughout your menstrual cycle, climbing four-tenths of a degree when you ovulate. Buy a basal thermometer (they cost less than $10), as it is more accurate than other types. It can be used in your mouth or rectum for the most accurate temperature reading down to a tenth of a degree. BBT must be recorded first thing each morning before you get out of bed. After a few months of charting, you'll see a pattern of highs and lows in the middle of your cycle, and BBT is at its highest point—around half a degree higher than normal—right after you ovulate. Subtle changes will occur when you're stressed, drink alcohol, are sick, use a heating pad or blanket, or get less than three hours of uninterrupted sleep, so make notes of any lifestyle factors that could impact your BBT. It's safe to have unprotected sex after the temperature increase is present for at least three days, but you must stop or use backup when your temperature drops again before your next period starts.

The cervical mucus method: The same hormones that steer your cycle also cause your cervix to produce mucus, which manifests as vaginal discharge. During different parts of your cycle, cervical mucus changes in color, texture, and volume. The changes are especially pronounced during ovulation. To try it, wipe the opening to your vagina before you pee and check the color and feel of the discharge on the toilet paper. You can also look at the color and texture on your underwear. If that doesn't work, put clean fingers into your vagina and rub the mucus between your thumb and index finger to feel the viscosity. Sex can change your cervical mucus, so avoid unprotected sex for at least one cycle while you're learning. What you're looking for is yellow, white, or cloudy mucus that is sticky, tacky, or slippery. That viscous texture helps sperm make their way to the egg, and the four days that mucus varietal is present are your most fertile days. After ovulation, there will be less mucus until your period begins.

Calendar charting: Basically, the rhythm method: track your cycle on a calendar or in an app for at least six cycles. You need a solid history before the data is reliable, and if your cycle is shorter than twenty-seven days, then this method will not be accurate enough to use without backup. Once you have six cycles of data, look for your shortest cycle, then subtract eighteen from the total number of days. Using a twenty-eight-day cycle as a reference, that is day eleven, which is your first official fertile day. The fertile window will be eleven days long, or until day twenty-two, which means during that time you must use backup or abstain. Yes, it is a long time, but unless you are also tracking your ovulation or BBT peaks, you will not know your true window for sure.

Efficacy: It's around 76 percent effective in pregnancy avoidance with average use. The full symptothermal method is difficult if you have gynecological conditions like PCOS that change cervical mucus consistency or cause delayed and irregular ovulation and irregular cycles. Other signs you have ovulated like spotting, mid-cycle pain or achiness (*mittelschmerz*—the Germans have a word for everything), increased energy, breast tenderness, and a heightened sense of smell, taste, or vision are useful to observe too. With all the these methods, pulling out is *not* a good backup.

Side effect: Unintentional pregnancy.

DIGITAL BIRTH CONTROL

Some period tracking apps have FDA-approved forms of contraception. They are marketed as hormone-free and natural and utilize many of the same data points of the fertility-awareness method. By ingesting months of tracked cycle data and running it through an algorithm based on millions of cycles, they can predict your fertile window. Usually, trackers are free with optional paid components. The algorithm is opaque—companies don't share how they determine fertility scores. And though the cost is relatively low, they are not reimbursable or covered by insurance yet. Digital birth control is still new and improving constantly with the vast amounts of data users are contributing, but most doctors warn that counting on it with no backup or abstinence during the fertile window is not a good idea, especially if you are sick or do anything else that could affect your BBT.

Efficacy: Companies claim it's around 92 percent effective for typical users; perfect use puts it closer to 97 percent. But there is a giant *but*: that efficacy number was determined in a controlled study with highly motivated, diligent participants who were closely tracked and compensated for their time. The real world is a little different, so many ob-gyns believe that efficacy is much closer to FAM.

Side effects: It's crucial in today's reproductive environment that you understand how and if the company sells, shares or anonymizes data to ensure your privacy, so read the terms of service. Otherwise, the only side effect is a more intimate relationship with your phone.

ABORTION

Abortion is the ending of a pregnancy—whether spontaneously as a miscarriage or therapeutically when a life-threatening condition during pregnancy occurs, or as a planned decision to terminate a pregnancy. More than 92 percent of planned abortions are performed in the first trimester, around 6 percent happen between fourteen and twenty weeks, and less than 1 percent are done after twenty-one weeks, almost exclusively to save the life of a pregnant woman or due to a fatal condition in a fetus. Regardless of why it happens, and which type is performed, abortion does not cause mental health problems or breast cancer and does not impact your ability to get pregnant in the future. There are two ways abortions are carried out: medically through a pill regimen, and surgically in a procedure known as a dilation and curettage (D&C), or, if later in pregnancy, a dilation and evacuation (D&E). All types are considered safe and rarely carry complications, and in the case of medical necessity, are far less risky than carrying a failing pregnancy to term.

Medical abortion is indicated until eleven weeks (or seventy-seven days) after the first day of your last menstrual period (or later in some countries outside the United States). Medical abortions can be obtained online through a telemedicine clinic or in an office. Telemedicine is only possible if you are eighteen or older, have regular periods, and have not had your tubes tied or a history of ectopic pregnancy. After you discuss your medical history and health conditions with a doctor or nurse practitioner, you will be prescribed two medications to take twenty-four to forty-eight hours apart: mifepristone swallowed with water, which blocks the release of progesterone, and misoprostol inserted vaginally or held between your cheeks and gums for thirty minutes. Misoprostol is a cervical-ripening agent also used during the induction of labor or to treat postpartum hemorrhage that causes uterine cramping and bleeding. You will not be sedated or need to go to a clinic—taking these pills can happen at home. The main risk with medical abortion is that sometimes it does not work fully the first time and requires a second round of treatment. Side effects can be heavy bleeding and cramping, and if you soak two pads per hour for two hours in a row, you should seek emergency care. Most symptoms like fever and chills, headache, nausea, vomiting, diarrhea, fatigue, and breast changes resolve in a few days. There are no blood tests for misoprostol or mifepristone, so if you present to the emergency room with bleeding and do not want to disclose you had a medical abortion, you do not have to. Your right to disclose is up to you, even when speaking with nurses and doctors, paramedics, and other healthcare personnel. If you decide not to disclose, you can say you are having a miscarriage, which is 100 percent accurate.

If you are past eleven weeks or are not a good candidate for medical abortion, you'll have a D&C. It is an outpatient procedure conducted in a doctor's office, or if you choose sedation, a hospital or outpatient surgery center. It starts with a cervical dilation, usually initiated by misoprostol (or a cervical dilator if you are past sixteen weeks). After your cervix dilates, a curette (a tube-shaped suction tool with a hole at the end) is inserted to scrape the endometrium and remove tissues. Abortion is not the only reason a D&C is performed. It can also be used to determine the cause of abnormal uterine bleeding; resolve a miscarriage, especially those where a fetus has died but the body has not miscarried naturally (a "missed" miscarriage); during infertility investigations, or to test for possible cancers. D&Cs are also sometimes used after childbirth to remove pieces of the placenta that remain attached to the endometrium. If you had an elective D&C and don't feel comfortable talking about it, again, it is your right to disclose whatever feels right for you, and it's fine to say that you had one to resolve a miscarriage.

So, does abortion hurt your fertility? A D&C is a surgical procedure, and the biggest risk is uterine perforation, occurring in fewer than two in one thousand women. There is an even smaller risk of developing a uterine infection. There are also rare cases of heavy bleeding, perforation of the uterine wall leading to bowel damage, and scar tissue inside of the uterus after the procedure, though these side effects happen to fewer than one in one thousand women. Whether medical or surgical, it's possible to get pregnant immediately after an abortion, so make sure you use contraception if that is not your intent. If you've had a D&C for any reason, speak to your ob-gyn about your circumstances and the timing. With medical abortions you can try again the next cycle, but after a D&C it's best to wait at least one full cycle and preferably two to three to allow your uterus, body, and mind to heal. No matter why you had one, abortions are emotional, so consider seeking support from friends or a therapist to process the experience.

I had a medically necessary abortion after a fatal chromosomal abnormality was discovered during my second pregnancy. It was the hardest experience of my life, and completely inconceivable to me that I would have to terminate a wanted pregnancy. That experience drove me to write my first book and engage in grief therapy to make sense of the whole thing. And it was not my last one either, as between the births of my two sons I had a missed miscarriage that did not resolve on its own. If the body does not miscarry naturally, there is a risk of sepsis. So mid-pandemic I went to the hospital by myself at 5:00 a.m. (no guests allowed, my husband had to pick me up curbside) for another D&C.

After going public with my experience, I know it is not often framed in this context. But abortions are not always a choice—sometimes they are a medical necessity. Miscarriages happen in as many as one in four pregnancies, so with that math even if you don't know about it, someone in your life has gone through a version of this experience.

STERILIZATION

Vasectomies

While it may not be on your mind currently, it's worth understanding long-term birth control options, especially since interest in vasectomies and vas occlusion (which involves a gel injected into the vas deferens that blocks sperm for up to a year) is growing. A traditional vasectomy shuts the ends of the sperm superhighway—the vas deferens—through a simple clinic-based procedure. The vas deferens is cut, sealed with heat, or blocked so that sperm cannot move from the testicles to the penis during ejaculation. The procedure is quick: the penis is held up or taped against the stomach; anesthesia is given; after the area is numbed, the vas deferens is clamped; and a urologist makes a small cut in the scrotal skin with a pair of razor-sharp scissors (it's numb! You won't feel it!), and a tiny piece of the vas is cut out and removed. Then the ends are sutured or cauterized, and the vas is returned to the scrotum, usually along with a bit of skin glue to close the miniscule cut.

If reading about a sharp implement near that body part stresses you out, you'll be happy to hear Valium and other anti-anxiety medications are sometimes given before surgery. There can be some pain in the first twenty-four to forty-eight hours, which is relieved with an ice pack (or frozen peas) and ibuprofen or acetaminophen, and slight swelling is a normal side effect. But other than taking a break from heavy lifting, exercise, sex, and masturbation for a week, that's it. Vasectomies are 98 percent effective but do not take you to sperm-zero immediately. Usually, it takes three months or around twenty ejaculations for sperm to disappear entirely. While OTC sperm count tests are useful to test the result, you'll get a more sensitive analysis in a follow-up appointment to know for sure if it worked.

Unlike tubal ligation, vasectomies are outpatient procedures with few complications and are far less expensive. They have no significant long-term health risks, and full recovery happens in about a week. Between 3 and 6 percent of men change their minds, and reversal success rates are between 60 and 95 percent in the first ten years and highest when the same physician that did the vasectomy does the reversal. Vasectomies are not a slam-dunk option for young men in their early twenties that want to conceive naturally later; it's more suited to those whose families are complete. If a reversal fails and there is no sperm found in your semen, there is an option to retrieve a sample and conceive via IVF: sperm aspiration from the testicles or vas deferens. If it's just a case of the sperm being unable to escape, this option works nearly 100 percent of the time, especially when done in conjunction with intracytoplasmic sperm injection (ICSI; a procedure that uses just one sperm to fertilize an egg during IVF). The sample isn't usually big enough to do intrauterine insemination (IUI). To future-proof your reproductive options (and it is increasingly part of presurgical counseling), consider putting some sperm on ice before a vasectomy.

Tubal ligations

Almost 19 percent of women claim to have had a sterilization procedure performed, and they are about five times as common as vasectomies for men. Usually this is performed as a tubal ligation, often referred to as getting your tubes tied; though many ob-gyns are recommending full removal of the tubes to prevent tubal or ovarian cancer. Tubal ligation is a misleading nickname as the procedure closes the fallopian tubes off with a ring, band, or clip, or cuts, clamps, or cauterizes them. It is a surgical procedure that starts with general anesthesia to put you to sleep and a few pumps of gas (carbon dioxide or nitrous oxide) via a needle or small incision into your belly to make your organs more visible. Then one or two small cuts are made near the belly button, and a laparoscope (a tool that features a light and camera) is inserted to find the fallopian tubes. When they are accessible, the tubes are cut or closed off, and the incision is sutured. There can be dizziness, nausea, cramps, or pain in your belly, but most people fully recover after a few days.

Even though tubal litigation is done laparoscopically or during a C-section for women whose families are complete, tubal ligations can result in vaginal bleeding and heavier periods for months afterward. Tubals that are done with clips and rings are more easily reversible, especially if there are still healthy fallopian tubes left post-surgery, but there is no guarantee. However, as with vasectomies, a failed reversal doesn't mean you cannot have a genetically related future child. Conceiving requires IVF, but it is usually possible to retrieve eggs directly from the ovaries and women with tubals can carry pregnancies. In fact, it's not uncommon for gestational carriers to have had a tubal ligation.

While failure rates for male and female sterilization are low, if you and your partner are trying to decide who should go under the knife, a vasectomy is less invasive, simpler, more effective, and can be more easily reversed if you change your mind.

BIRTH CONTROL DETOXES

Innumerable influencers advertise that hormonal birth control requires a special detox. *Their* special detox plan, as it happens. And it sounds plausible, right? Pulling the goalie seems like it needs a recovery plan, especially if you've been on hormonal birth control for a decade or more. But only one form (the shot), has a longish return to normal fertility. Between nine and thirteen hours after you stop oral contraceptives more than half of the pill is completely undetectable, and remember that it is possible with most forms of birth control to get pregnant one cycle after you stop. Ninety-seven percent of women return to a normal menstrual cycle within ninety days of dropping the pill, and within one year, 87 percent of oral contraceptive users are pregnant. There are side effects from dropping the hormones that range from irregular periods, moodiness, acne, and hair loss to sudden rage at your partner for not doing the dishes.

There can be less obvious changes too, for example, hormonal birth control made with estrogen treats acne, so you may need to reinvest in a new skincare regimen. But these hormone imbalances do not last long, and for most people, no action beyond letting your body find its new normal is required.

The concept of birth control detoxing is popular because it is believed that taking it "masks" symptoms of other conditions. While this is technically correct, that's the point of using birth control as a therapy. The pill can help treat symptoms of PCOS but does not hide enough symptoms to block a diagnosis from being made. Conditions like PCOS have genetic and environmental influences, not just one underlying cause, and it takes more than one symptom to diagnose it. The pill cannot fix all of them. But as mentioned previously, when left untreated, PCOS and other gynecological conditions can cause anovulation. So if you notice any new symptoms when you quit, take note, and talk to your provider. Even if you decide to start a detox, pay close attention to how your body changes and your new point of stasis first.

Birth control detoxes generally entail a mix of lifestyle guidance and supplements to rebalance your hormones. If you pursue it or a specialized return to fertility program, like analyzing research studies, consider the source. Ask yourself if this information is coming from a company or human with a financial upside. Is what they are saying based on real science? Real science means clinical studies published in reputable journals performed with true rigor, or literature reviews showing data combined from multiple studies, totaling thousands of people tested. Some of these protocols and supplements do work for people but probably not for the reasons we think. Often they suggest common sense, healthy guidance—like practicing moderation—and staying away from endocrine-disrupting chemicals, eating whole foods, and avoiding added sugars and trans fats, not smoking, and moving your body alongside their custom supplement regimen. So it's easy to believe that the positive result is because of the pills instead of the lifestyle changes that really fuel these improvements.

Birth Control Wrap-Up

- The "right" birth control is a balance between what works best for your life and what matches your fertility goals.

- No forms of hormonal birth control have permanent effects on your fertility. The shot is the only one with a more than transient delay— between five and eight months.

- The pill is not the only hormonal birth control option: there are rings, shots, patches, implants, and IUDs.

- FAM and the symptothermal method are great ways to get to know your cycle in preparation for TTC, but they are not foolproof forms of contraception.

- Basal body temperature and cervical mucus can be difficult to monitor if you have some gynecological conditions, and both are impacted by lifestyle factors like alcohol intake and sleep.

- If you feel unsure about your ability to understand cervical mucus or forget to chart your BBT frequently, FAM and digital birth control should be accompanied by backup birth control methods, especially during your fertile window. It can also be helpful to use an OPK.

Hearing that there aren't proven mood-related side effects to hormonal birth control felt like total BS to me too. During my first month on the pill at seventeen I ran my car into a parking lot post and burst into tears. I found myself crying frequently, over nothing in particular too. It took three different formulations—estrogen, combo, and finally the progestin-only pill that I am still on today—to find one that worked. After several decades on that pill, I quit so we could TTC and found myself enraged over household slights like not doing the dishes (sorry, Nick). In contrast to many people's experiences, I am a happier, saner, more balanced person with better skin on birth control. But even with my freak-outs, there was no delay back to normal fertility. We were pregnant the cycle after I stopped taking the pill.

Part 2

Optimizing Fertility

Chapter 6

NUTRITION AND GUT HEALTH

How what you eat and weigh influence fertility

Homo sapiens began our reign on earth as hunters and gatherers. The earliest iteration ate like chimps, foraging on fruits, flowers, bark, insects, leaves, and meat. Traveling in small nomadic groups, they didn't mingle often with one another. Then the world changed. The rise of crop cultivation and domesticated livestock made accessing food more predictable, and humans began to live as larger groups in fixed geographies. But it came at a cost: our symbiotic relationship with nature and its microbes changed, as did our diets. Easier access to animal protein, transitioning to life in urban settings, and exposure to pathogens and zoonoses changed the collection of bacteria that lives in our gut, and not for the better. Later in 1896, Professor Wilbur O. Atwater sealed a graduate student in an airtight chamber and watched him eat precisely measured servings of milk, mashed potatoes, and steak. The chamber was a calorimeter, and it quantified the amount of heat the energy in the food generated through the chemical reactions and physical changes it catalyzed in the student's body. Atwater concluded that eating is governed by mathematical laws, and thus the calorie was born. From that moment on, calories dominated diets, conversations, and nutritional policy. Governments were thrilled, as it gave them a way to quantify nutritional needs in schools, prisons, and army bases, and the food industry was forced to adopt it to communicate a product's role in today's one-size-fits-all, generic two-thousand-calorie-per-day diet.

Our relationship with food today is more convenient than any other time in human history, and the unhealthiest. Most of the world eats a highly processed diet sans good fat, fiber, and enough vitamins and minerals. Our ancestors ate foods that came from the ground; now food is pumped out of machines into bags and boxes and packed with preservatives to help its shelf life last a year or more. Livestock are bred and fed to optimize their size and speed to market and are less healthy than the versions our grandparents ate (never mind the cruel conditions rampant in factory farming). The famously lean chicken now has nine times more fat than previous iterations when commercially grown. Our sedentary lifestyles, noxious food sources, and yen for convenience mean that most people's diets are in some way out of whack. And the result can be dysbiosis, or a lack of microbial diversity in our guts, which is associated with chronic inflammatory diseases that impact fertility. The concept of food as medicine lives exclusively in the wellness world unless a nutritionist is part of your care team, as future doctors receive just twenty hours of nutrition instruction during medical school and rarely broach the topic later during appointments. Unlike other areas of fertility research that are squishy at best, we know a lot about the impacts of food, and they are meaningful. But it's not as simple as eating salmon, nuts, and berries.

While there are vitamins and minerals associated with a fertility-friendly diet, there are problems with today's aggressively prescriptive approach. The first: what we eat is not just about nutrition or basic survival; it reflects our values and priorities. Dietary choices are dictated by our preferences and cultural and religious traditions, which winnow the menu of available options. If you are strongly against factory farming, for example, there is nothing anyone can say to tempt you to eat chicken unless, perhaps, you can source it locally. Each person's nutritional requirements, which change based on activity, biology, genetics, and many other factors, are also different. Glycemic responses to the same foods can be totally distinct from person to person too.

The weight-loss industry is now worth a staggering $300 billion despite the fact that diets, cleanses, and detoxes do not work over the long term. There is no evidence that weight loss supplements work either. The only diet with clinical evidence showing somewhat improved fertility is the Mediterranean diet, but even there, the study's sample size was small and only observed couples going through IVF. Diets are frameworks to help make better, more consistent choices, and we should refocus on other aspects like the quality and quantity of the foods we eat. Our bodies are programmed to digest and use whole foods, not highly processed substances thrust out of drive-thru windows. Because our bodies don't intrinsically know how to process these foods, the more we eat them, the more our hormones change unnaturally to accommodate them.

A LIGHT CONVERSATION ABOUT WEIGHT

Healthy bodies can look very different, so what follows has nothing to do with aesthetics. But here is the difficult truth: an unhealthy weight, no matter the circumstance or why, dramatically impacts the ability to conceive and support a pregnancy—and it cuts both ways. Women who try to conceive with a high body mass index (BMI) take twice as long to get pregnant and have high-risk pregnancies and deliveries. Obesity also negatively influences a baby's brain development, cardiac activity, and motor skills. Conceiving with a low BMI is difficult too, as being underweight can cause anovulation. Underweight women take four times as long to conceive as those in the healthy range.

Let's talk about BMI for a moment, as it is a lazy, flawed way to sort humans into health categories, but is still the way your physician will talk to you about your weight. Created to understand communities, not individuals, BMI is a calculation of your weight in kilograms over your height squared in centimeters. Its inventor, Adolphe Quetelet, was an academic trying to quantify the weight of the average human at a population level. His formula was derived from data on white, mostly male Western Europeans, so it does not reflect or accurately measure people of color or women. BMI only diagnoses obesity correctly 50 percent of the time and detects less than 50 percent of obesity in Black, white, and Hispanic women. BMI also misses the effects of a more muscular frame, as muscle is 80 percent water and heavier than fat, which contains just 5 to 10 percent. A critical input to understanding a person's overall health excluded from BMI calculus is *where* they carry weight. Depending upon fat's location, even for those in the normal category, whether it's found around the hips, butt, or stomach can indicate increased risk for conditions like heart disease and diabetes. There are big differences in the way men and women gain weight too. Men carry it in their waists while women gain on their hips and thighs. A better way to create an overall health assessment is a hip or waist measurement or by measuring walking speed.

No matter how it is measured, the negative effects of being clinically overweight or underweight on fertility are caused by the body's stores of fat, which bring about hormone imbalances. Adipose tissue, or body fat, is found under the skin, around internal organs, between muscles, in breast tissue, and within bone marrow. Body fat is an important endocrine organ, and these cells play important roles in hormone production, metabolism, and regulation. Fat cells contain adipocytes, or cells that store and release energy throughout the human body, and others that produce hormones, regulate glucose, cholesterol, and metabolize sex hormones. Levels of fat in the body influence everything from puberty, sexual maturation, brain function, sleep, and fertility to lipid storage and energy metabolism.

The most well-known diagnosis for those with too much adipose tissue is obesity. It is a complex and serious disease caused by excess fat that can cascade into type 2 diabetes, high blood pressure, high cholesterol, and increased risk of blood clots, which taken together form a condition known as metabolic syndrome. Though it is primarily diagnosed via BMI, doctors also look at vital signs like blood pressure and heart rate, and physically examine the abdomen.

Obesity is one of the top causes of infertility for women, as it has a negative impact on ovulation, conception, implantation, and fetal development, and causes endocrine conditions like PCOS, which can make it difficult to maintain a healthy weight. A higher than normal body fat percentage changes the quality and potency of estrogen, can convert androgen, usually testosterone, into estrogen, and changes the function of sex-hormone-binding globulin, which is responsible for accurately transporting androgens and estrogens to the right tissues around the body.

Men are affected by obesity too. Obese men have lower testosterone levels and poorer quality sperm that can be traced all the way back to the germ cells in the testes, as they too are physically and molecularly abnormal. Male obesity impairs the metabolic and reproductive health of future children through this affected sperm. Couples with two obese partners take longer to conceive and are sometimes unable to conceive at all. People with high BMI often face discrimination in healthcare settings, and bias with infertility treatment. If you fall into this category and are having difficulty conceiving, but not long enough to see a reproductive specialist, reducing your weight is the recommended first step. However, the issue that is preventing pregnancy could be completely unrelated to weight, so if nothing is working on the timeline to seek care, insist on fertility testing or do a hormone panel on your own.

A lack of adipose tissue causes fertility problems in those diagnosed as underweight. Studies suggest women need 26 to 28 percent body fat to maintain a regular menstrual cycle and ovulate. Athletes and dancers who fit the normal BMI category due to their musculature can still have amenorrhea simply because there isn't enough fat to regulate hormones. Without a period, there is usually no ovulation, which makes getting pregnant impossible. For men, the effects of low

BMI on fertility and semen parameters haven't been studied enough to say anything conclusively, although the existing body of research indicates it decreases sperm count and semen volume, and impacts its overall quality. If you fall into this category and cannot gain weight or are struggling with disordered eating, make a nutritionist part of your care team, as an underweight BMI also negatively impacts pregnancy.

Most people believe weight is dictated solely by calories in, calories out. But some scientists now think that it may be more related to a dysregulated hormonal and metabolic response to the carbohydrates in our diets. A framework known as the carbohydrate-insulin model posits that the quality and quantity of carbohydrates we eat changes our hormonal functioning, which then contributes to the accumulation of excess fat. Calories are, like BMI, a flawed way to dictate our diets as they do not account for the quality of a food or factors like satiation. And all of the above is why, ultimately, eating a balanced diet packed with whole foods benefits everyone.

BUILDING A SUSTAINABLE, LONG-TERM FERTILITY DIET

You probably get it at this point: fad diets do not lead to long-term weight loss, or improved health over time. Highly restrictive fertility diets often make people eat more, and caloric restriction increases cortisol and can mess with other hormone levels too. Couples who diet together have more successful outcomes; though hormone and body composition are different for men and women, so plans will not be identical. Men's testosterone levels are ten times higher than women's, and women are more sensitive to caloric and carbohydrate restriction, which can trigger amenorrhea and inflammation.

Most nutritionists and behavioral psychologists suggest following the 80/20 rule, meaning 80 percent of the time you follow a healthy nutritional plan and the other 20 you explore less healthy foods, while being mindful and moderate in your choices. If you want more structure, use a food-tracking app or write down meals, or take photos of what you eat so you can review portion sizes and a meal's composition. The purpose is not obsession, it is to understand the rhythm of your natural behaviors and to help set a new baseline and habits. Over time, our brains associate certain foods with emotions, like ice cream with comfort. These habit loops become automatic and unconscious, so when we don't feel great, we reach for something we think will make us feel better. The only way to break the cycle is to think about why you're eating that food, reminding yourself that food cannot fix how you're feeling. Mindful eating is also critical, so slow down to think about how full you are before you start, take longer to chew, savor your food, and reflect on how you feel afterward.

Now, on to the reason you're here: the nitty-gritty of fertility-friendly eating and all the details around specific nutrients and foods.

Nutrient Basics

Carbohydrates	**Eat more:** Whole grains (bulgur, brown rice, oats, farro, quinoa, and millet) and fruit.
	Eat less: White carbs (white rice, bread, pasta, pastries, desserts, and cereals) due to added sugars and high glycemic index.
Fat	**Eat more:** Monosaturated fats are healthy and necessary; no need to pursue a low or no-fat diet. They are found in oily fish, olive oil and other plant-based oils, avocado, nuts, and seeds, which are fine in small amounts.
	Eat less: Processed foods that contain trans fat or polyunsaturated fat.

Protein	**Eat more:** Fish, lean meat, eggs, legumes, and dairy, which are all good protein sources, as are plant-based proteins found in grains like quinoa, or unsweetened Greek, Icelandic, and live yogurts.
	Eat less: Too much red meat can hurt your fertility (especially sperm), so keep steak and burgers as an occasional treat.
Dairy	**Eat more:** There is no proof cutting dairy entirely is necessary for your fertility unless you have issues digesting it (and many of us do). Some lactose-intolerant women can eat hard cheeses, and it is a good source of calcium. Be reasonable with your cheese consumption and try low-sugar Greek yogurt, as it is packed with protein.
	Eat less: High intake of low-fat dairy may increase anovulatory infertility and reasonable lactose consumption may not affect it at all, so stick with full-fat products. The reason: when the fat is skimmed from milk, the estrogen and progesterone are removed, and all that remains is the fat and testosterone. Without the fat to balance the sugar, the sugar ratios in milk are higher and contribute to insulin issues.

CHOOSING THE MOST FERTILITY-FRIENDLY PROCESSED FOODS

Nutritional labels didn't exist before 1973, as there were fewer food manufacturers and products on grocery store shelves, so there used to be zero transparency into what was in processed foods. It wasn't until 1990 that the FDA proposed a set of daily reference values to help consumers make more informed choices. The nutritional label is based on a generic two-thousand-calorie-per-day guideline, even though the appropriate number should be individualized based upon activity level, size, goals, and general health. Pertinent to those looking to use calorie count to lose weight, labels can also be inaccurate. The FDA requires that the calories, sugars, total fat, saturated fat, cholesterol, and sodium all be 120 percent or less of their actual total. That's right: if a label says an item is five hundred calories, and a lab analysis reveals that it is six hundred calories, the label is still considered compliant. Labels also indicate the serving size, which may surprise you, as even small bags of snacks can contain more than one serving. For the manufacturer, the goal is a size that feels sufficient for consumers but allows the package to keep other nutritional elements within the bounds to qualify it as a healthy option.

Processed foods are now 57 percent of all foods consumed in the United States and comprise 70 percent of options on grocery store shelves. Trans fats and added sugars are the two key items found on nutritional labels that you should avoid for your fertility and overall health. Fast foods contain large amounts of both. Though the research is less conclusive, artificial sweeteners may be just as problematic as added sugar. All the foods that contain these ingredients are ultra-processed, and come clearly marked with a nutritional label, so they're easy to spot. The other big problem with processed foods, which we'll cover in depth later, is the added exposure to plastics and other chemicals that drive our hormones wild.

Trans fats

Your body needs fat to survive—20 to 30 percent of your daily calories to be exact—but it does not need the trans fats found in fast foods and grab-and-go snacks. Small amounts of trans fats are also found in meat and dairy products from cows, sheep, and goats, and are fine in moderation. If you're choosing a product that contains trans fats, minimize consumption with any partially hydrogenated or hydrogenated oils listed on the ingredients list.

How do they impact fertility? Every 2 percent increase in calories women derive from trans fats versus other carbs leads to a 73 percent increase in ovulatory infertility. A pre-pregnancy diet packed with trans fats also puts you at increased risk for gestational diabetes. For both sexes, artificial trans fats raise LDL (bad cholesterol) and lower HDL (good cholesterol), which leads to build-up in your arteries, a leading cause of heart disease and stroke and other serious health conditions.

Found in fast foods, packaged and frozen foods (pizzas, ice cream, frozen yogurt, pudding), fried and battered foods, baked goods like cakes, pies, doughnuts, shortening, crackers, chips and other snack foods, margarine, nondairy creamer, and processed vegetable oils.

Added sugars

The average American consumes around sixty pounds of added sugar per year. It is a form of refined sugar added to packaged goods to make them taste better. Sugar is not inherently bad for you—your body needs some as an energy source. But humans were not biologically designed to digest processed additives, just sugar in the form of fructose from whole fruits.

How do they impact fertility? Sugar-sweetened beverages and snacks are correlated with lower fertility for men and women. Drinking just one soda each day reduces the odds of conceiving in a year by 20 percent. They negatively affect sperm parameters, and women who consume them have higher risks of infertility. Added sugars can also lead to insulin resistance, fatty liver disease, and increased triglyceride levels, elevating your risk for heart disease.

Found in fruit juices, smoothies, soda (if you care about your fertility stop drinking it), energy drinks, packaged snacks, sweetened tea and coffee drinks, candy, desserts, and baked goods (cakes, cookies, pies), sauces (ketchup, barbecue sauce, salad dressing), crackers, and some yogurts. Look at the ingredient list for items that end in -ose (dextrose, fructose, glucose, lactose, maltose, sucrose) or juices, nectars, and syrups. Common types of added sugars are agave, cane sugar, raw sugar, turbinado sugar, corn syrup (including high-fructose corn syrup), maple syrup, honey, and cane juice. Some are marketed as "natural" but are no better nutritionally than cane sugar.

**Artificial
sweeteners**

Artificial sweeteners were invented by the food industry to satiate our collective sweet tooth without the calories of real sugar. Since artificial sugars don't trigger the same satiety mechanism in the brain, they can cause weight gain, which runs counter to their reputation as a weight-loss product.

How do they impact fertility? Artificial sugars may alter metabolic pathways and induce glucose intolerance. Daily diet soda consumption is associated with a higher risk of metabolic syndrome and type 2 diabetes, conditions that negatively impact fertility. Women who consumed drinks containing artificial sweeteners during an IVF cycle had decreased egg quality, embryo quality, and reduced implantation rates. Men experience negative effects on their sperm parameters, including more DNA fragmentation. During pregnancy, consuming one to four artificial sugar-powered beverages per day increased the risk of preterm delivery even after controlling for confounding factors.

Found in diet soft drinks, powdered drink mixes, baked goods and snacks, candy, canned foods, jams and jellies, pudding, and dairy products. Products that are labeled "sugar-free" or contain aspartame, saccharin, stevia (it's derived from natural ingredients but is still refined), sucralose, and tagatose.

THE TRUTH ABOUT ALCOHOL AND CAFFEINE

Bad news for men who love beer and cocktails: too much alcohol lowers testosterone levels and hurts sperm parameters like count and quality. If you've ever tried to have sex after one too many drinks, you know that it can also cause issues getting or keeping it up and with ejaculation, and it decreases libido. Long-term, heavy alcohol use in men is also associated with testicular atrophy, liver dysfunction, and azoospermia. Low to moderate alcohol drinkers, meaning fewer than fifteen drinks per week and no more than two per day, do not generally have these problems. However, men who drank even moderately in the month before and especially the same week as sperm collection for IVF cycles were less likely to achieve a live birth.

For women, drinking while you're in conception mode is tricky because of the two-week delay between ovulation and the possibility of getting a positive pregnancy test, though an accidental rager before a missed period will not cause any lasting harm. If it had, the pregnancy would have ended as a very early miscarriage before you knew you were pregnant. Fetal alcohol syndrome is caused by heavy drinking during the entirety of a pregnancy—not a one-time event. That said, the data on alcohol is all over the place, as most is self-reported, and people fudge the numbers when they feel embarrassed. Alcohol is a known teratogen (birth-defect-causing substance) and the period when things are most likely to go wrong is the first trimester. Drinking during pregnancy at all is not recommended, but especially important to avoid during the first twelve weeks, when the baby's core organ systems are forming. Because a pregnancy begins before you have any way of knowing you are pregnant (most tests can only accurately test starting in the fourth week), it's safest to just cut consumption after your big shot on goal.

The data we have on low and moderate pre-pregnancy alcohol consumption does not seem to correlate with increased risk of miscarriage or stillbirths, though it also relies on self-reported data. There is some proof that binge drinking can affect egg quality, though research has only been done on mice. Egg growth and maturation takes months, and repeated heavy exposure to alcohol has been shown to affect the development of follicles and the body's ability to accurately perform cell division during early embryo development. During IVF, you'll be told to keep alcohol consumption very low or preferably stop. Drinking alcohol has secondary effects like inhibiting hunger and satiety hormones and fat oxidation, and makes your body store more fat, which is another consideration before you pick up a second (or third) glass.

Better news, coffee lovers. Repeated studies show that moderate caffeine consumption does not negatively affect pregnancy, nor does it hurt female fertility. Moderate means keeping your total daily consumption under two hundred milligrams of caffeine per day, which is equal to two small cups of brewed coffee. Don't forget to include other sources of caffeine—teas, sodas (soda is not part of any fertility-friendly diet, so if that is how you are getting your caffeine, switch to coffee or tea), aspirin, energy drinks, and chocolate in your calculation. Caffeine temporarily increases blood pressure and heart rate, and acts as a diuretic, which for some people is a plus while others don't appreciate the sudden, urgent trips to the loo. For men the evidence is still mixed. Some studies show that the same moderate consumption is good for sperm while others say too much decreases sperm quality.

FERTILITY POWER FOODS

If you go all in on a fertility-friendly diet, the foods below have a combination of the right vitamins and minerals, folate, fats, carbs, and fiber for your everyday diet, and clinical evidence shows some improvement to fertility. For example, Vitamin D deficiencies cause fertility issues for women and men, and combined with their omega-3 content, make salmon and other oily fish fertility superfoods. Sunflower seeds provide a boost thanks to their combination of fatty acids, folate, and selenium. Oranges and grapefruit contain vitamin C and polyamine putrescine, which is associated with improved egg and semen health. Watermelon is known as "natural Viagra" for its aphrodisiac qualities and help with erectile dysfunction. PCOS sufferers who supplement with cinnamon have more frequent menstrual cycles and improved ovulation. Creating a diet that excludes everything else isn't necessary, and not all of these foods will fit everyone's preferences, so stick to whole, unprocessed foods as your guiding principle and try not to obsess.

Berries	Eating fruit improves pregnancy rates, but some choices are more fertility-friendly than others. Bananas (especially very ripe bananas, which are the fruit equivalent of candy bars), grapes, mangoes, pineapple, and dates are all heavy on sugar but light on fiber, which can cause blood sugar spikes, so enjoy sparingly. Berries—blackberries, blueberries, and raspberries especially—are full of nutrients like fiber, vitamin C, iron, and B vitamins, packed with antioxidants like anthocyanin, and lower in sugar. Blueberries win for overall fertility friendliness, but all berries are great snack choices.
Oats	The base of fertility power breakfasts (or whatever time of day pleases you) is the reliable, malleable oat, thanks to its fiber content, low glycemic index, and blood sugar friendliness. Studies done on IVF patients show oats and whole grains improve implantation and live birth rates, and the impacts are assumed to be similar for natural conception. Cinnamon and berries add sweetness without sugar or try a savory version with the spice of your choice.

Eggs	Choline needs during pregnancy impact everything from placental function to a baby's brain development, and it reduces the odds of developing neural tube defects or chronic diseases. Research on choline is new, so not all prenatal vitamin formulations include it. Luckily, choline is found naturally in animal products, especially eggs, and dairy, chicken, beef, and salmon, and soybeans. Most people don't get enough, so diversify your diet before you start TTC.
Leafy greens	Kale, spinach, romaine, and collard greens are the most fertility-friendly greens, and the winner is kale, with 25 percent of the daily folate requirement in one cup. If you're not into raw foods, greens can be cooked, steamed, sauteed, roasted, combined into other dishes, or served on top of brown rice.
Oily fish	Though they are packed with a strong smell and taste, oily little anchovies (easily hidden in pasta sauces) are low in mercury unlike some of their fishy counterparts, rich in the omega-3 fatty acids DHA and EPA, and a healthy source of fat proven to decrease inflammation and insulin resistance. Wild-caught salmon is a similarly lauded fertility protein; it contains the same marine omega-3 fats. Filets should be a vibrant orange color, not pale pink.

Nuts	Sunflower seeds have a perfect combination of fatty acids, folate, and selenium. Almonds are packed with folate and come in sweet or savory flavor profiles. Three Brazil nuts each day meet the daily requirement for selenium, which is essential for thyroid function and DNA health, and protects cells from damage by free radicals. Salted nuts contain loads of sodium, so opt for other seasonings or unsalted versions. Nuts are healthy when not coated with sugar but are dense and contain many calories. A serving size should be ten almonds or less.
Quinoa	It looks and tastes like a grain, but surprise! Quinoa is a seed. Pronounced "keen-wah," it has been a staple food in Bolivia and Peru for five thousand years, where it's believed quinoa improves the quality of breast milk. Full of protein and fiber, quinoa contains high levels of iron, magnesium, and zinc. For anyone with dietary restrictions, it is gluten-free and low on the glycemic index and good at any meal, from breakfast with nuts and fruit to savory dishes like stuffed peppers or in place of rice.
Legumes	Easy to add to most savory dishes, chickpeas are a great source of fiber and folate, and good for your gut. Black beans reign supreme on folate content, making them an excellent option. Lentils are high in protein and fiber and low in fat while containing folate, iron, phosphorus, and potassium.

Fermented cabbage	Whether you are at a beer hall or Korean barbecue, fermented cabbage is commonly in the form of sauerkraut or kimchi, and like its leafy green cousins, full of folate. Fermented foods are good for your gut, and boost microbiome diversity and immune responses, so as a bonus try kefir, miso, and sourdough breads (sourdough starter is a live, fermented culture of flour and water).
Avocado	Avocados are fruits, not vegetables. They hit high marks for the triple combination of monounsaturated fats, fiber, and folate, and vitamins B and E. Avo can be smeared on toast, added to a salad, or eaten alone with a bit of salt and sesame seeds or sumac.

FERTILITY-FRIENDLY COOKING OILS

We already lauded the Mediterranean diet, but here's another reason to make the primary oil in your life plant-based, or more specifically, olive oil. Studies show that people who consume olive oil versus animal fats like butter have lower risk of cardiovascular disease, cancer, neurodegenerative disease, and a slew of chronic diseases. Those in the highest echelon of olive oil consumption, which is more than seven grams per day, have the most risk-lowering benefits versus those who never or rarely consume it. The benefits extended to other plant-based oils too. While olive oil consumption has not specifically been tied to fertility, hopefully you get that the healthier your body is overall, the better your fertility is too.

Plant-based oils are extracted from seeds and nuts through a press or crushing process. If the label says "virgin" that means it is unrefined and has not undergone processing outside of that initial extraction.

The only downsides are that virgin oils do not have a neutral flavor profile (you can't use them for everything), they retain minerals and enzymes that don't do well with high heat, and tend toward rancidity more quickly than other choices. Virgin oils are best used to make salad dressings to drizzle as a finisher, and for low-temperature cooking. Oils with high smoke points, or the temperature at which they stop shimmering and start smoking, undergo manufacturing processes like bleaching, filtering, or high-temperature heating to eliminate troublemaker enzymes and ingredients. When an oil is pushed past its smoke point, it releases free radicals and acrolein, a chemical that lends an unsavory acrid flavor to foods and will fill your kitchen with smoke.

Coming in at the top of the smoke-point spectrum are avocado oil, the number one fertility-friendly choice, and safflower oil. Both start smoking around 510 to 520 degrees Fahrenheit/270 degrees Celsius. Light and refined olive oil, soybean, peanut, and sunflower clock in around 450 degrees Fahrenheit/230 degrees Celsius and all have a neutral flavor profile. But importantly, they feature omega-6 oils, not the omega-3s found in salmon that are more fertility-friendly. If you're searing, neutral fats with a high smoke point like peanut or corn are good options. Deep frying is best left to safflower and peanut, both of which can take high heat. And for sautéing, which doesn't need to be blazing hot, extra virgin or light olive oils are excellent choices to impart flavor.

COOKING HACKS FOR THOSE WITH ZERO TIME OR INTEREST

Between trips to the grocery store and cooking, preparing meals can be time intensive, and not everyone enjoys it. But it is the easiest and best way to know exactly what you are putting into your body. To get over the hump, here are a few practical tips to make cooking less painful.

Plan your meals for the week: Look at your calendar and see how many meals you need to have on hand that week. Make a grocery list and order or pick up ingredients just once or twice that week, depending on how many of the fresh items will go bad.

Use grocery store delivery services: All major cities and most rural areas have teams of shoppers and delivery drivers ready to help you avoid trips to the grocery store or allow you to order ahead and pick up on the way home from work. The cost is little more than doing it yourself, and saves many hours over time.

Keep recipes simple: No one needs a multicourse, James Beard Award–worthy meal every night. Select easy recipes and high-quality ingredients that taste good on their own. Look for recipes that can be made in a single pot or on a sheet pan, like fish and vegetables, or soups and stews, and require little attention.

Cook in bulk: Rather than cooking five dinners during the week, cook two or three and eat the leftovers. Choose recipes that are easy to scale up and store well (keep dressing and salads separate to avoid sogginess). If your food muse calls, prepare and freeze multiple meals so they're ready to pop into the oven.

Consolidate your cleanup: Facing a giant pile of dirty dishes after dinner prevents a lot of people from repeating the effort. Use a large mixing bowl to gather (and compost if you can) food scraps and optimize for simple recipes that can be cooked in one pot or on a sheet pan and clean up as you go.

Make your kitchen a place you enjoy: Invest a small amount to make your kitchen a cheerful, happy, organized place that is nice to be in even when you aren't cooking. If you plan to cook more often, purchase good tools like sharp knives and cookware, as sharp knives counterintuitively reduce the likelihood you will cut yourself.

Still not into cooking? Prepped boxes are here for you: If you can't find your kitchen zen, no problem. There are boxes of prepped fresh ingredients that come to your front door ready to mix and cook or reheat (don't microwave food in plastic!). To select a good one, read about their ingredients and recipes and look at nutritional information. Most cost the same as or less than takeout.

TO DETOX, OR NOT TO DETOX?

The theory of the diet detox centers around the idea that your body is full of accumulated toxins, heavy metals, and inflammation that needs to be purged, usually through fasting or herbs or specific diets. Our bodies are constantly exposed to unnatural chemicals through food and the environment, and studies have shown over and over that everyone benefits from eating organic diets, as it lessens exposure to pesticides used in agricultural production, reducing endocrine disruption. But a cleanse cannot erase a lifetime of exposures, and hardly anyone can, nor should they, adhere to one for a long period of time. There is some evidence to support short-term benefits and healthier levels of toxins in the body, but if you revert to old behaviors, it all comes back. That's why the biggest long-term benefit of a cleanse or detox is the reset it gives your body and mind, pointing you toward mindful eating so you pay attention to what you put into your body long after it concludes.

If a reboot sounds good, here is how most fertility cleanses and detoxes work. They come in kits, weeklong and monthlong plans. Some are led by practitioners, and most of the focus is on the uterus and liver, both of which need to be in healthy working condition when a pregnancy starts. If you're a fan of Chinese medicine, the goal is to increase blood circulation to the reproductive organs, tonify the uterine tissue, and help normalize the menstrual cycle if it is irregular. This treatment path requires working with a practitioner who will tailor a specific regimen to your body and needs in concert with your other health providers. Options may include herbs like white peony for hormone balances, red raspberry tea, nettles, and other compounds. We'll cover the wild world of supplements in the next chapter, but a warning: they are largely unregulated in the United States, meaning they have not gone through the same level of FDA regulation as pharmaceuticals and can have powerful positive and negative effects in the body. Many herbs for fertility are contraindicated for pregnancy or interact with other medications. If you're pursuing fertility treatments it is crucial to be upfront with your doctor about other practitioners you are seeing and all herbs and medications you are taking. Fertility cleanses and caloric restriction should not be done within six weeks of trying to conceive, and preferably end even further in advance so your menstrual cycle is unaffected. Continuing to take herbs or cleansing while pregnant is a big no unless (and this is unlikely) it is clinically indicated, and you are under the care of a provider who is monitoring you.

Time-boxing a period to avoid unhealthy or processed foods and focus on your health is great. Keeping healthy habits after that period concludes is the goal. And this little adventure does not have to come in the form of a pricey soup cleanse or brew of herbs. Simply following a high-protein, low-carb, organic diet that features healthy fats and whole foods has clinically validated positive effects on fertility.

LESS OBVIOUS BUT IMPORTANT ASPECTS OF MAINTAINING YOUR GUT HEALTH

Balancing your blood sugar

If you feel blah in the middle of the day or right after a meal, blame a blood sugar dip. Though the terms are used interchangeably, insulin, glucose, and blood sugar are not the same thing, and each has a different role in powering your body. Glucose is the sugar that comes from the foods that you eat. It is your body's primary energy source and becomes blood glucose or blood sugar when it travels through your bloodstream to power your cells. Insulin is the hormone that makes this travel possible.

Diabetics have high levels of glucose in their blood because they either do not have enough insulin to move it to their cells or their cells do not respond to insulin as they should. More than 180 million people around the world have diabetes, and there are two types. Type 1 usually appears during childhood, and though we don't know for sure, it may be caused by genetics or exposure to viruses or other environmental factors. Type 1 diabetics do not produce enough or any insulin to allow glucose to enter cells and produce energy. There is no cure for type 1 diabetes, so it takes active management to prevent complications. Type 1 diabetes is associated with DNA fragmentation in sperm, and for women can lead to irregular and longer cycles, anovulation, and the production of antibodies that attack sperm and eggs. Type 2 diabetes happens when the insulin your body produces does not work the way it's supposed to. While it historically affects postmenopausal women, with rising obesity rates, it is now common during the fertile years too. Women with type 2 diabetes are more likely to have PCOS. It can create poor semen parameters for men, especially sperm concentration and motility, and increased DNA fragmentation. And the world's number one drug to treat type 2 diabetes, metformin, is now associated with genital birth defects for the sons of those men who took it in the three months before conception. So, if you have diabetes, talk to your doctor, and if it's possible, especially for men, control your blood sugar through diet and lifestyle if you plan to conceive.

Managing your blood sugar can cause problems with your fertility even if you don't have diabetes. Sugary diets and those high in empty calories, processed fats, and flours cause blood sugar crashes. Skipping meals is a trigger for your body to go into survival mode, increasing your cortisol levels. Insulin resistance happens when the cells in your muscles, fat, and liver don't respond to insulin and cannot use glucose to power your body. The result is that your pancreas makes more and more insulin to help your cells absorb glucose. PCOS, obesity, and physical inactivity are all contributors to insulin resistance. While there are many tests to diagnose diabetes, there isn't one for insulin resistance. A healthy diet, weight loss, and increased physical activity can help your body respond more appropriately to insulin. Short sleep duration is a risk factor for obesity and causes blood sugar fluctuations. When poor sleepers slept an extra 1.2 hours per night their daily energy intake dropped by 270 calories. This is not surprising, as the body produces more ghrelin (the hunger hormone) and less leptin (a hormone that helps with satiation) when you are sleep-deprived, making you feel like you need to eat more.

Identifying food allergies and intolerances

If your digestion is out of whack and you can't figure out why, it may be a food allergy or intolerance. So, what's the difference? Food intolerances cause digestive issues several hours after eating. They usually go away on their own (though they can be very uncomfortable) and are not life-threatening. Food allergies can cause life-threatening symptoms like trouble breathing or skin reactions in addition to digestive issues and happen immediately after eating every time you consume a particular food. They also cause major quality-of-life issues, and disrupt fertility, putting people at increased risk of delayed conception, miscarriage, and disturbed menstrual function.

Food allergies are easier to diagnose than intolerances. If your reactions are serious, find an allergist or book an appointment with your primary care provider for a referral. If it's just the occasional annoyance or you're curious, order a simple food tolerance test to take from home. Allergy testing can rule out allergies, but not guarantee that you have one. A standard skin test is done one of three ways: a prick or puncture that scratches the skin so a tiny bit of a specific allergen can be introduced; intradermal skin testing where the allergen is injected under the top layer of the skin; and patch testing, where the allergen is put on the skin for two days to see if there is a reaction. Blood testing for IgE antibodies to specific allergens is another method, which happens in a lab with a phlebotomist or via tests you order online. If you do it yourself, you submit the sample via a dried blood spot, using a lancet to prick your finger and catching drops of blood on a card that you mail to a lab for analysis. If you are allergic to specific foods, the antibody levels will be high, indicating an immune response. But even with higher-than-normal levels of reaction to certain foods, an allergy is not a certainty, as the presence of other conditions like eczema or asthma can elevate them as well.

Food intolerances do not show up on tests, and sometimes the underlying food itself isn't to blame—a specific ingredient, preservative, or additive is. Though a hydrogen breath test can help to identify some food intolerances, an elimination diet accompanied by a food diary is the best way to identify problem foods. Make a note in your phone or use an app to track everything you eat for two weeks. Note any time that you have a bad reaction, then look for patterns, and at the end of your two weeks eliminate the foods that trigger you one at a time for two weeks each (no overlapping). If eliminating that food helps without making any other changes, you are likely intolerant. Common culprits are dairy and gluten but can be more subtle, like dairy products that contain lactose. If it's more serious, your care team will grow to include a gastroenterologist, as conditions like inflammatory bowel disease, celiac disease, and hemochromatosis are associated with infertility and early miscarriage. Undiagnosed celiac disease, for example, can be present in women with unexplained subfertility or recurrent miscarriages, yet it is not often tested.

Diversifying your gut microbiome

The body's microbiome is made of trillions of microorganisms consisting of thousands of microbial species including bacteria, fungi, parasites, and viruses. These busy microbiotas live in a delicate balance throughout the body, and play diverse roles in its daily operation, from stimulating the immune system to synthesizing vitamins, and protecting the body from pathogens. A human's original set of microbes is inherited from their mother, via the birth canal and breast milk. Throughout life, environmental factors and diet transform its makeup. The body has many microbiomes—oral, vaginal, and nasal among them—but the most studied is the gut. This field of study is called nutritional psychiatry, and it examines the connections between what you eat and how you feel based on the colony of bacteria, fungi, and microbes that control digestion and parts of the immune system. While around 6 percent of the microbial species in the gut are inherited, 48 percent are explained by cohabitation, or where we live and who we live with. Gut microbiome composition changes with diet and stress levels, sleep, exercise, and lifestyle factors. Early studies show that more diverse gut microbiota may be attributed to higher fertility for women. It can also affect response to cancer therapy, from melanoma to lung and kidney cancer. One study done on post-acute COVID-19 syndrome patients showed that six months after recovery their gut microbiomes were markedly different from the controls. There are multiple links between mental health and the microbiome too, most famously depression.

For all its promise, we do not fully understand the gut microbiome, making the landscape of tests and diagnostics interesting but not terribly useful yet. The old-fashioned method—a food diary—is still the gold standard for identifying food triggers and improving one's diet. We have yet to unravel what an optimum microbiome is, or if that standard is even the same for everyone. The exact microbe species can vary widely from person to person and still comprise a healthy microbiome. Geography and environment have roles in determining a person's basic microbial makeup too. Like most of health, scientists believe that it's highly personal and more about having the right balance of bacteria than a universal standard.

Nutrition and Gut Health Wrap-Up

- Eat real, unprocessed whole foods as often as you can. Bonus points if you buy organic meat and produce when you're able.

- Be mindful of what you are eating and pay attention to your body's cues. Portion size matters, and frequent unhealthy snacking between meals can set back all your hard work.

- Perfection is not a reasonable goal for most people, so strive for 80 percent adherence to a good diet, and 20 percent of the time eat what you want (without bingeing).

- The Mediterranean diet is a good template: whole grains, lean protein, and healthy fats. More specifically fresh vegetables, oily fish, poultry, and moderate amounts of fresh fruit (not juice!).

- Read nutritional labels and stay away from trans fats, added sugars, and artificial sweeteners.

- Sodas and other sugar-sweetened beverages cause insulin spikes and should be avoided.

- Find ways to enjoy occasional cooking or use a grocery delivery service to keep healthy food around.

- Make meals in bulk and freeze or try healthy meal delivery services.

- Fertility cleanses aren't permanent solutions; think of them as a reboot to start healthier long-term habits.

Starting in my mid-twenties, I had severe, debilitating gut issues. At the time it felt random—there was no telling what food would set me off. When I sought treatment, my symptoms were brushed off as PMS for over five years. Finally, I found a gastroenterologist who believed it might be a bigger issue and one colonoscopy later I was diagnosed with ulcerative colitis, a form of inflammatory bowel disease (IBD). While it was a relief to feel heard (and less crazy), that day my life changed drastically. Medication and a completely new way of looking at my diet shifted how I looked at food forever. After hearing stories from other patients, my goal became managing my condition through diet so I could someday stop medication. After a year of tracking everything I ate in a food diary, trends emerged. Cow's milk (especially ice cream, which I love), fried foods, arugula (I don't get it either), and red meat had to go. But a decade later, I am still in remission, and medication-free. IBD is associated with an increased risk of miscarriage, so I am glad I dealt with my issues before conception and had the tools to manage it. Also, during pregnancy, some of my trigger foods (in small portions) didn't bother me, so I was able to even enjoy ice cream for a few blissful months.

Chapter 7

SUPPLEMENTS

Pills are not a panacea—how to use supplements correctly to maximize fertility

The term "vitamine" was coined in 1912 by Casimir Funk. While studying beriberi (thiamine deficiency), Funk realized that the Asian populations who suffered from it most ate a lot of polished rice and that the issue was the absence of a nutrient rather than the existence of a toxin. And thus, the study of deficiency diseases, which are curable with vitamins, began. In 1916, Mastin's yeast Vitamon Tablets became the first mainstream multivitamin. The formulation was a potent concoction of vitamins A, B, C, calcium, iron, and nux vomica, which is derived from strychnine. Promising pep and clearing the skin, it claimed to aid digestion, correct constipation, and improve the appetite. The *Journal of the American Medical Association* (JAMA) was not pleased with this product or those that followed, stating, "The claims set forth on the labels of the medicinal values of these preparations are extravagant and misleading." It was the first of many hot takes from the medical establishment, which is still skeptical of the benefits of supplements. Some of their concern, as you'll learn, is for good reason.

The human body does its best absorption of vitamins and minerals when they are packaged together in food; they are not meant to be taken in isolation. Eating healthy whole foods is the most effective way to ensure your body gets what it needs. While the first generation of vitamins was extracted from food, now ingredients are made in labs, including those labeled as "food state" or "whole food," and many contain synthetic elements and artificial additives. The starter culture food-state vitamin C, for example, is lab-synthesized ascorbic acid. Too much of a single vitamin or mineral leads to expensive pee, as most of the time the body cannot absorb excess levels and eliminates the rest. Some specific fat-soluble vitamins and nutrients can also lead to overaccumulation and serious issues like liver toxicity. Taking the wrong supplement can cause problems too. The Selenium and Vitamin E Cancer Prevention Trial (SELECT) study concluded far before its deadline when scientists figured out that supplementing with high doses of vitamin E increased prostate cancer rates instead of reducing them.

Three out of four American adults take a dietary supplement thinking it will radically transform their health. The value of the supplement industry reflects it and is now worth more than $150 billion and set to grow to $250 billion globally by 2028. The appeal is simple: What could be better than a magic, all-natural substance you pop into your mouth that fixes fertility (or frankly, anything else)? It's an easy way to make you feel like you're doing something, which is a powerful proposition if you're struggling with infertility.

Homeopathic medicines are another subset of the supplement category and are a popular way to "naturally" improve fertility. Like supplements, homeopathic treatments are not well regulated, and many have active ingredients that do more harm than good especially when not taken as directed.

Some supplements do fill a real need, as most people do not get every single nutrient they need even from a diverse, healthy diet. And those considering conception should absolutely take a prenatal vitamin three months or more before they start trying so folate levels have a chance to build up.

Supplements in the United States are regulated like food, not drugs, so adverse effects are found only after demonstrated harm has occurred. The argument for keeping the industry this way is that running herbs and dietary supplements through the same vetting process as pharmaceuticals would put them financially out of reach for most people and limit the number of manufacturers who could produce them. But the lack of regulation also means that some products are found to be contaminated with heavy metals, contain ingredients that are not listed, have doses that are higher or lower than what is stated on the packaging, or have serious interactions with other medications. There is no independent organization checking these safety parameters for the public. Safety information is not available even if you do want it—there is no requirement to test new products and ingredients before marketing them—so consumers don't have a clue how potentially dangerous supplements can be either. From Hydroxycut, with its links to liver damage, to ephedra, which was tied to stroke and heart arrhythmia, there is a long list of supplement recalls due to health problems and death discovered only after they hit shelves.

POPULAR FERTILITY SUPPLEMENTS

There are a growing number of supplement makers promising to improve your fertility with their special formulation. In the throes of infertility, if someone offers an easy solution (or really, any solution), most people click Buy without thinking about it. But before you waste your money, the evidence on most supplements is mixed at best, as the category has not been studied enough, and nearly all options you find on Instagram are not endorsed by your reproductive endocrinologist or ob-gyn. Beware of claims by a single or a few doctors hyping the bona fides of specific supplements; those are paid ads. Even the evidence on supplements like antioxidants for men, which have few side effects and are frequently recommended, is low quality. When it comes to fertility, you should exercise even more caution, since side effects and interactions are poorly understood. Make sure any supplements you take are appropriate for you or your partner and use them only as directed. While nothing listed here has known serious side effects, it's important to speak to each physician who is treating you for other conditions, especially if they are prescribing drugs. Even though many come formulated as gummies, supplements aren't candy—each comes with superpowers that can cause interactions, side effects, or make other conditions worse. If you're a fertility supplement wonk, you'll notice that for women, evening primrose oil and chasteberry are not included. The reason: both have known interactions with other drugs and require more research to understand when they are indicated and if and why they work.

Common Fertility Supplements for Men and Women

A high-quality prenatal vitamin (or multivitamin for men)	A prenatal vitamin taken three months (or longer) before you plan to conceive is the only universally recommended fertility supplement for women. Folate, or vitamin B9, is the key ingredient and will appear on packaging as folic acid, the synthetic form. Folate occurs naturally in foods like eggs, leafy greens, avocado, and liver, and refined grains like cereal, flour, and pasta are enriched with folic acid. Every prenatal vitamin must contain four hundred micrograms of folic acid, iron, calcium, vitamin D, iodine, omega-3 fatty acids (DHA and EPA), and choline.
	If you have a MTHFR gene mutation, as 30 to 40 percent of people unknowingly do, your body cannot properly convert or absorb folic acid. This mutation is associated with hormonal changes, digestion, cholesterol, brain function, and may be a cause of recurrent miscarriage (though evidence is mixed).

Carriers of this mutation are usually asymptomatic, so routine testing is not required. The problem no longer exists when you choose a prenatal made with the active, methalyzed form of folic acid, 5-MTHFR.

Side effects are minimal, but the iron in prenatals can cause constipation, nausea, and other gastro issues, so take them before bed or with a snack or find a food-based version that is easier to digest.

While it's not essential for men, taking a prenatal or high-quality multivitamin falls into the category of does no harm. Folate helps make blood cells, DNA and RNA, converts carbohydrates into energy, and is a key ingredient in sperm development. Today's male prenatal vitamins contain a cocktail of the ingredients below like coenzyme Q10, DHA, lycopene, selenium, and vitamins C, D, and E, all of which have evidence of improved male fertility.

What it helps: Taken during pregnancy, it is proven to reduce neural tube and heart defects, preterm birth, low birth weights, and even the risk of autism. Taken any time it may help with anovulatory infertility and improve rates of conception in women undergoing IVF. For men, low folate levels are associated with lower sperm quality and concentration and increased DNA fragmentation.

| Coenzyme Q10 (CoQ10) | The most proven and highly regarded fertility supplement for both sexes, CoQ10 is a nutrient that is made naturally in the body and stored primarily in the mitochondrial cells, heart, liver, kidney, and pancreas. It is found in many foods and provides energy to cells, ⇨ |

Coenzyme Q10 (CoQ10) (*cont.*)	is essential for metabolism, and acts as an antioxidant, protecting our cells from damage. Ubiquinol and ubiquinone are the two active ingredient options. Ubiquinol is touted as the active form of CoQ10 and more bioavailable, meaning your body absorbs it more easily. But it can be unstable in supplement form, and studies that show benefits are based on ubiquinone. **What it helps:** Mitochondrial function drops as we age, and that drop is correlated with decreased ovarian reserve and premature ovarian aging as well as maternal mitochondrial genetic disease. CoQ10 enhances mitochondrial activity, and since its levels also dip as we age supplementation for those older than thirty-five is recommended. For women, it also improves egg quality and quantity and pregnancy rates, and is helpful in combating age-related fertility decline. For men, it boosts sperm motility, concentration, and counts as well as fertilization rates.
N-acetyl-cysteine (NAC)	NAC is an antioxidant and an FDA-approved drug used to treat acetaminophen poisoning. Its other association is with unexplained fertility, but NAC may have insulin-sensitizing properties too. We think NAC might help induce ovulation, and when tested during IUI cycles, it significantly improved pregnancy rates without ovarian hyperstimulation. Due to its role as an antioxidant, NAC may improve sperm parameters. **What it helps:** For women, it may help with unexplained infertility or problems related to ovulation. For men, it improves sperm count and motility, DNA fragmentation, and protamine deficiency.

Selenium	Selenium is a mineral that naturally occurs in soil, water, and some foods. Whether alone or combined with vitamins C or E or folate, it is a well-regarded fertility supplement for men. Semen with lower levels of selenium and zinc is correlated with poor sperm quality. Studies show that three months of a combination of selenium and vitamin E for men with low sperm count and motility may improve spontaneous pregnancy rates by nearly 11 percent. For women, its antioxidant superpowers help promote healthy uterine follicles.
	What it helps: For both, thyroid function. For men, sperm count and motility. For women, possibly egg quality.
Vitamin D	Human skin produces vitamin D naturally after exposure to UV rays. Its most famous role is to absorb calcium, but it also helps with cell growth, immune response, and controlling inflammation. Over half the world's population does not get enough vitamin D because we mostly live indoors these days and wear sunscreen when we play outside. But it's also a function of air pollution in some parts of the world. Having enough vitamin D in your blood is associated with higher pregnancy and birth rates whereas having an insufficiency may lead to first-trimester miscarriage as it can impact embryo development.
	What it helps: For women, it increases the odds of conception and success during IVF, reduces the risk of miscarriage, and supports immune function and bone health. For men, it improves overall semen quality and sperm motility.

Zinc	Zinc is a trace element and nutrient that helps with immune and metabolic function. Found in red meat, poultry, and fish, the human body cannot make zinc. Zinc is especially important for men, as spermatogenesis and testosterone are affected by its levels. Poor zinc status is a risk factor for low sperm quality and male infertility. For women, dietary zinc availability is a key factor in female egg development, and zinc deficiency is also tied to epigenetic defects in eggs. **What it helps:** For men, sperm morphology, motility, and volume. For women, egg quality.

Supplements Just for Men

Ashwagandha	Used in traditional Indian Ayurvedic medicine as an aphrodisiac and treatment for male sexual dysfunction and infertility, one study showed that Indian ginseng, or ashwagandha, increased sperm counts by 167 percent, motility by 57 percent, and semen volume by 53 percent. There are also compelling early studies that show an improvement in stress and anxiety levels and improved sleep, making it a popular wellness supplement. **What it helps:** Sperm count, motility, volume.
Lycopene	Responsible for the rosy hues of guava, watermelon, tomatoes, and papaya, lycopene is a natural compound found in foods. In the American diet, it's mostly consumed as cooked tomatoes in pizza sauce and ketchup. But even in that format, it is an

antioxidant that fights free radicals that cause cell damage. One study showed that supplementing with twenty-five milligrams of lycopene for twelve weeks increased total sperm count and concentration along with ejaculate volume and motility.

What it helps: Sperm count, concentration, motility, and ejaculate volume.

Supplements Just for Women

Dehydro-epiandrosterone (DHEA)	If you have diminished ovarian reserve (DOR), this is a good supplement to consider. But it has only been shown to improve pregnancy rates in those with DOR—it is not a fertility super pill. DHEA is a prohormone, or a hormone that makes other hormones like testosterone and estrogen, and during IVF is linked to higher follicle counts, more eggs retrieved, and lower medication requirements. **What it helps:** For women with DOR, it may boost pregnancy rates and help with egg count during IVF treatments. It is not proven to help those with normal ovarian reserve or women going through an egg freezing cycle.
Myoinositol	This is a popular supplement with midwives, especially to help prevent gestational diabetes. And while it's officially called vitamin B8, it's a type of sugar found in nuts, beans, fruits, vegetables, and grains. It shows promise in improving egg and embryo quality in PCOS patients, as it may help ⇨

Myoinositol (*cont.*)	normalize ovarian function. Myoinositol decreases LH and androgen as well as insulin resistance, and can induce ovulation, making it a tool to reestablish regular ovulatory menstrual cycles. The impacts on pregnancy rates are less clear. It still falls into the category of promising, as most trials are low quality to date and were conducted on assisted reproduction industry (ART) patients, but we know enough about the mechanisms that it is worth considering. Myoinositol is low cost and does not carry any known side effects, so if you have PCOS or diabetes, speak to your provider about it.
	What it helps: Corrects the LH/FSH ratio, reduces androgen levels, can help reestablish regular ovulatory cycles, and reduces insulin resistance for diabetes and PCOS patients.

CHOOSING THE RIGHT SUPPLEMENT FORMULATION

Supplements aren't just tablets and capsules—they can be powders, chews, gummies, and liquids too. When a manufacturer creates a supplement, choosing the optimal delivery format is a question of how to best deliver the required serving size of ingredients in the most user-friendly and convenient method. There are physical limitations to how much of one vitamin or mineral can be crammed into a single tablet or capsule, which is why some formulations require taking two or three or even more to achieve a single serving. While some people dislike swallowing that many pills, most don't mind gummies, which is why gummies account for over 10 percent of the supplement market today.

The two-piece hard-shell capsule is the oldest and most common format because it allows a rapid release in around ten to fifteen minutes and doesn't require as many processing aids. Made of animal-derived gelatin or plant-based cellulose or pullulan, its physical transparency lends that attribute to our perception of the product itself, since we can see what's inside. Depending upon the formula, tablets and some capsules offer more variety in shape and size. This allows the ingredients to be time-released in closer to thirty minutes, although they can be larger and harder to swallow. You'll find soft gels for formulas that are liquid or oil-based, like fish oil. Powders are ideal for supplements that require a large serving size but must be dissolved in liquid. Many also require processing excipients to stop them from clogging up machines during processing, to avoid clumping in storage, and to improve their dissolvability. Gummies hold appeal to kids and adults who hate swallowing vitamins but include added sugars. The other downside of gummy supplements is that they do not always contain the nutrient levels required to be effective. When sugars, coloring, and filler compounds are required to make a texture work, there isn't always room. Before you buy, check the company's website for information on sourcing, quality assurance, and the formulation to ensure it contains the correct percentage of different nutrients.

If you're a vegetarian, the word *gelatin* may pop out. Many supplements, especially capsule shells, contain gelatin, a protein made from boiling animal skin, tendons, ligaments, or bones in water. If a supplement is plant-based or vegetarian, it is usually indicated on the packaging. Finding a gummy formulation that does not contain gelatin can be a challenge, as it is the primary coagulant for most commercially successful brands. Pectin and agar are more difficult to work with and result in a less traditional texture but meet the vegan requirement. Many gummies also contain gluten, dairy, and high-fructose corn syrup. Overconsumption is a common problem (especially for kids and adults who view them as candy) and puts you at risk of getting too much of some nutrients, which in rare cases can end in vitamin or mineral toxicity. Unless there is a good reason to consume your supplements as a gummy, pick a tablet or capsule instead. Regardless of delivery format, always follow the dosing and ensure that if you are taking more than one supplement, they don't contain overlapping ingredients. Quality matters, so only buy from reputable companies. You'll know they are reputable if you look for information about the traceability of their supply chains and how they source ingredients, as many now advertise these processes.

SUPPLEMENTS ARE GREAT, BUT CANNOT FIX EVERYTHING

Judging by the appetite for supplements you'd assume they work miracles. In the case of the prenatal vitamin, the positive results are proven. But in some cases, the effects are more psychological than biological, a phenomenon known as the placebo effect. Placebos are sham substances designed to have no therapeutic value, but they sometimes cause a therapeutic effect anyway because our brain thinks they should. During clinical trials there are even placebo surgeries where patients undergo an imitation of an entire procedure, from the fasting and anesthesia to the recovery room, but not the procedure itself. A review of this unbelievable practice showed that sham surgeries provide some benefit in 74 percent of trials and work as well as real surgeries in over half. Whether we are susceptible to the placebo effect can come down to genetics, as there appear to be variations in the brain's neurotransmitter pathways that make it more or less likely to work. The belief that expensive supplements are more powerful than cheaper versions is a prime example of the placebo effect.

Supplements cannot treat serious disease or deficiencies. However, they are cheap relative to most of Western medicine, and when used correctly, can provide health benefits while tricking our brains into thinking we are more in control. That benefit alone can drive down cortisol levels, especially during an infertility journey. Little money goes into supplement research, though more is happening now since vitamin D, zinc, and others were used in the management of COVID-19 in hospitals. Some supplements have European Food Safety Authority (EFSA) approved health claims because there is a body of evidence for specific formulations used at specific dosages to justify it. But the two supplements you can feel great about for women and men based on their strong evidence are the marvelous prenatal and CoQ10.

During my struggles, I was ad-targeted nonstop by fertility companies and influencers who promised to fix my problems with their bespoke formulations or programs that cost hundreds and sometimes thousands of dollars. After researching these protocols, many lacked any scientific basis, and if they did have scientific basis, relied primarily on changing lifestyle and dietary habits. Targeting someone facing fertility problems with pseudoscience knowing they will do anything to make a baby is predatory and really pisses me off. There are great companies and people in the mix, but finding them requires diligence.

Supplements Wrap-Up

- The only supplement that is mandatory for women is a prenatal vitamin, preferably started three months before TTC. Men can take a high-quality multivitamin or prenatal too.

- Supplements cannot fix your fertility—they can only fill deficiencies in your diet or lifestyle.

- Supplements are not the ideal way to get vitamins and minerals. Change your diet and eat more whole, unprocessed foods first if you have nutritional deficiencies.

- Purchase supplements from companies with good sourcing practices and a commitment to high quality ingredients.

- If you are taking any medications, work with your provider before taking any supplements to ensure there are no adverse interactions.

- Supplements backed by evidence for men: CoQ10, a prenatal formulation containing a mix of Vitamins C, D, E, folate, zinc, and selenium, or a multivitamin is also great.

- Supplements backed by evidence for women: A good prenatal vitamin that contains enough folate, CoQ10, zinc, and NAC. DHEA and Myo-Inositol work only for specific conditions.

Chapter 8

EXERCISE

How activity can boost your fertility and prepare your body for pregnancy

The ancient Greeks were first to formalize specific exercises and physical training for men who competed in the Olympic Games. Women had their version
of the Olympics too—the Heraean Games. They served as a warm-up to the
Olympics, and events were run on shorter courses with an emphasis on agil-
ity. Exercises that focused on power or endurance were the dominion of men,
as it was understood even then that strenuous exertion negatively impacted
the menstrual cycle. There was also a fear that being hit in the uterus would
leave a woman unable to conceive. While this is rarely a concern preconception, during pregnancy a direct hit to the abdomen can cause everything from
placental abruption to miscarriage and is why contact sports are discouraged.
After the Romans banned the Olympics in 394, claiming they encouraged
paganism, organized exercise among civilians mostly died out until the games
restarted in 1896. The only other group with formalized training regimens was
the military. Outside of fame, fortune, and glory, the goal of a male fitness
routine was to stay in shape and have attractive body proportions and musculature for procreation purposes. While the desirability of specific body shapes
has remained pretty consistent for men through the millennia, the perceived
attractiveness of women's bodies could fill a book. Just in the past forty years

we've gone from bodysuit-clad fitness fanatics doing calisthenics in the 1980s to pin-thin waifs with protruding bones and no breasts in the 1990s, to the big booties of the 2010s and back around again.

The earliest humans didn't block their calendars for fitness classes or leave home to throw heavy weights around at a gym. Nor did they exercise to fit an ever-changing ideal body type. A basic level of physical activity was part of life, as most walked five miles or more daily performing basic functions like hunting and gathering food. The idea of deliberately exercising to improve one's health is recent, since food procurement now is less chasing animals and plowing fields and more ordering groceries that automagically appear at the front door.

Nearly all forms of physical activity are good for male and female fertility. Moving your body helps improve mental health and can reduce cortisol levels too. Obesity is a fertility killer for both sexes, and exercise helps weight maintenance and loss. However, exercising too intensely can also hurt fertility, leaving you without enough adipose tissue to regulate your hormones. Moderation is key, and activities that fall into a chill category are still great, even if it's a quick thirty-minute stroll around the block. If your job involves a lot of time in front of a computer, try not to sit too much, and make any call you can a walking call. Men, that means you too—lethargy is no good for sperm. Neither is your cycling habit.

Humans are designed to move. Our springy arched feet and short toes are adaptations that help us walk and run more efficiently. Yet even with an abundance of data disproving it, many women believe that exercising before trying to conceive and during pregnancy is a no-no. If you still think that's true, it may be because fifty years ago doctors told their patients that exercise could make them barren, and like birth control, these myths take a long time to correct. Men are told nothing about the impact of exercise on their fertility even though it has a big effect on sperm. Watching too much TV hurts sperm concentration and count, and doing just thirty minutes of moderate exercise three times a week can improve those same parameters. Working out too hard can cause anovulation for women and low testosterone levels in men, but regular moderate exercise improves just about everything. Even relatively small doses of physical activity are good for your mental health, as adults who walk briskly two and a half hours per week have a lower risk of depression, and exercisers have fewer days of poor mental health overall.

At the risk of being a broken record, maintaining a healthy weight is one of the best things you can do for your fertility. A high BMI is associated with too much body fat, which throws off hormone levels. A low BMI also causes problems, primarily a stop to ovulation for women and lower testosterone for men. If you're pursuing IUI or IVF, a normal BMI increases the chance of having successful assisted reproduction treatments too.

EXERCISING BEFORE AND DURING PREGNANCY

The rumor that women who exercise too much will be barren persists because of the impacts on ovulation, and anovulation is the cause of around 30 percent of female infertility. But PCOS, not overexercising, is the cause of 80 percent of anovulatory infertility, and moderate exercise reduces symptoms for PCOS patients. A review of studies done on exercise and ovulation showed that heavy exercise, defined as more than sixty minutes of strenuous, heart-pumping activity per day, may disrupt ovulation while vigorous exercise between thirty and sixty minutes per day is less associated with anovulatory infertility. We think that the mechanism that impacts ovulation is the modulation of the hypothalamic-pituitary-gonadal (HPG) axis, which we know as the body's stress-response alarm system and manager of cortisol levels. Light and moderate activity reduces the risk of most other ovulation problems too and later during pregnancy, miscarriage risk.

There's another big reason for women to begin exercising before conceiving. Pregnancy is physically (and emotionally) taxing, and going through it with a strong body makes the experience easier. It can also prevent postpartum pelvic floor dysfunction like incontinence, which is experienced by 33 percent of women. That number is likely low since pelvic floor conditions frequently go undiagnosed and untreated. Strong abdominals help with pushing the baby out, and may facilitate faster recovery from cesarean births and conditions like diastasis recti, which persist in 60 percent of women during the postpartum period. Activity benefits babies too. It protects them from developing metabolic problems even with a high-fat maternal diet. Infants born to mothers who exercised during pregnancy had better motor skills and cardiovascular function too.

The official recommendation is that all adults between eighteen and sixty-four years old get 150 minutes per week of moderate-intensity physical activity. Today's options are endless, and the goal should be finding an activity you enjoy that best serves your body. Pilates, yoga, swimming, and walking are all well-known fertility-friendly activities. If that's not your jam, there are many others, and one activity that may surprise you. Only 20 percent of women do any form of strength or resistance training, as there is an assumption that it makes you bulky or the time isn't worth the effort (it doesn't, and it is), but strength training is a great option even into pregnancy. For men, pretty much everything is on the table with one exception. Even low-intensity cycling negatively impacts every single semen parameter, so stop at least thirty days but preferably three months before you TTC to allow your testicles to recover. If cycling is your passion and you can't quit entirely, there are noseless seats to better accommodate your testicles. But even then, it should be at the bottom of the list of physical activities to pursue before conception.

WHAT DOES MODERATE EXERCISE MEAN, ANYWAY?

The advice to pursue "moderate" activity sounds easy enough, but really, how do you know? The short answer is, it's personal, and what is intense to one person might be easy for an elite athlete. As usual, the medical establishment is here with another framework to determine each person's perfect level. The Borg scale of exertion was invented to answer this question by a Swedish researcher named Gunnar Borg in 1998. Borg realized that while humans are built to do various types of physical activity and work, too much or too little can be detrimental, and defining that level of output with purely physiological measures like heart rate and VO_2 max didn't paint the full picture. He felt that a qualitative scale would be the ideal complement, allowing providers and fitness professionals to understand individual clients based on their own feedback. The Borg Rating of Perceived Exertion (RPE) uses a scale that runs between six and twenty (one to five are basically sitting still), with six equaling watching television and twenty finishing the last leg of an intense race, and asks exercisers to self-report how hard an exercise feels. Multiplying that perceived exertion level by ten should be about the same as the heart rate. Moderate exercise on Borg's scale is between twelve and fifteen, which on the top end is around 150 beats per minute. If you work with a physician or trainer with a clinical background, this may be how they frame it.

If this sounds too complicated or you don't want to wear a heart rate monitor, try the talk test. It's how physicians suggest pregnant women calibrate their exercise and works well for anyone, anytime. It's simple: if you can talk through an exercise and aren't so winded that words are tough to choke out, you're working out at a moderate level. If you stay at a heart-pounding pace and cannot talk, you are in the intense-exercise category and should slow it down. Duration wise, if conception is imminent, keep your workouts, especially anything close to strenuous, to under an hour at a time.

FERTILITY-FRIENDLY ACTIVITIES

Going to a fitness class is a fine way to exercise, as is a brisk walk. If you prefer to sweat privately, there are connected devices and apps that fit into a corner of your home. From smart rowers and reformers to bikes and strength-training setups, they integrate with your other devices and fit more easily into a busy schedule. Booking even a single session with a personal trainer can be helpful to put together a plan, whether by video or at a studio. If price or storage space put those out of reach, there are apps that provide asynchronous workouts with a few simple pieces of equipment that you can stash under a bed, or thousands of classes online that use only body weight.

Many people rely on group fitness classes or a workout buddy or personal trainer for the social pressure. If your feelings on exercise are ambivalent, ask yourself what feels good and why you're exercising. If it's for fun and enjoyment or finding a connection to your body, amazing. If what you're doing isn't working, or you dread every second, consider what you want to accomplish and on what timeline and change it up. Recruit a friend! If you're trying to lose weight, some exercises are better than others. Losing one pound requires burning thirty-five hundred calories, which is more than you'll achieve in any single fitness class or workout. Increasing your caloric intake alongside exercise will make you gain weight. Like a healthy diet, a good exercise routine is a long-term, sustainable commitment that (hopefully) grows into something you enjoy.

BUILDING THE OPTIMAL FERTILITY-FRIENDLY EXERCISE PLAN

If you are starting a new routine, or are new to exercise, talk to your doctor before jumping in—especially if you have a chronic condition or are trying to conceive. To kick you off, here are a few tips all personal trainers and physical therapists wish people would follow regardless of the activity they are pursuing, from beginners to experienced athletes.

Don't go too hard too fast

Starting a new routine is exciting, but if your body isn't used to much or any activity, you're more likely to get injured. Intense activity that comes out of nowhere can negatively jolt your muscles, heart, and joints. Instead, start with light- or moderate-level exercise, then add time and more difficult movement types as you progress over a few weeks or months.

Warm up and cool down

It may not be the most exciting part of an exercise routine but taking a few minutes to warm up and cool down increases the likelihood that you stay injury-free and will improve the quality of your workouts. Light movements like arm circles or neck stretching or foam rolling help to loosen your muscles and joints and initiate blood flow throughout your body. To cool down, slow down whatever movement you're doing to allow your heart rate to drop. After it has, do a few deep stretches of the areas that you worked to help with recovery. Beyond protecting against injuries, it will decrease muscle soreness the next day. Neither must be long—five to ten minutes is all it takes. And there is no right way—target the muscles and areas that feel most fatigued and hold each pose until you feel the area release.

Stay hydrated

If you live in a hot climate or high altitude, this is especially important. Drink water—that's it. No fancy sports drinks promising to restore your electrolyte levels. Most have close to your daily sugar allotment and zero nutritional content. Unless you are an elite athlete or doing something truly strenuous (and hey, we're not doing that, right?) it isn't necessary. Drink a minimum of twenty-four ounces of water per hour of moderate exercise, during or after.

Plan exercise during your peak energy hours

With everything else we have going on, it's easy for exercise to fall by the wayside. Intent and follow-through is everything when establishing new habits, so work it into your day in a way that feels sustainable. Enlist a buddy or trainer if you need extra accountability. What time of day you exercise can determine the strength and type of metabolic response too. Your circadian clock is responsible for biological processes like metabolism, hormone production, immunity, and behavior. And it's all communicated to the body via light exposure. Exercise timing rewires intra-tissue and inter-tissue metabolite correlations, and whether it's done early in the day or later in the day changes the function of some of our organs and metabolism. We can't say definitively whether working out in the wee hours or early evening is better, as each carries different benefits, so it's best to do it when your life allows.

Exercise with the phases of your menstrual cycle

There may be no universally perfect time of day to move your body, but for women, we know that the body responds to activity uniquely through the menstrual cycle as different phases are associated with varying energy levels. If you're ready to tune in, you can synchronize specific activity types with menstrual cycle phases. A cycle-friendly routine optimizes for the best output at each phase. Using a textbook twenty-eight-day cycle as a template, the menstrual phase (days one through seven) is for gentle exercise, follicular (days eight through thirteen) is for more intensity, ovulatory (days fourteen through twenty-one) is for heavy weights, then it's time to dial things back during the luteal phase (days twenty-two through twenty-eight).

MEET YOUR PELVIC FLOOR

Greetings, and meet the important area of your body that you may not even know exists: the pelvic floor. If you're wondering what or where exactly that is, your pelvic floor is the bowl-shaped set of muscles that support your uterus, bladder, and other internal reproductive organs. You can think of it as a muscle hammock that stretches between the tailbone and pubic bone in the pelvis and helps regulate your bowel movements, urination, and sexual function while physically support-ing those critical organs. During pregnancy it will support the weight of your growing baby, which makes going into pregnancy with a well-functioning pelvic floor doubly important. Most people don't think much about this muscle group, even though it is connected to many others, until something goes wrong.

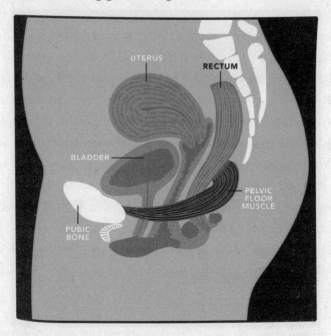

More than half of women will experience a pelvic floor problem at some point in their lives, and 11 percent will undergo surgery for related issues. After childbirth, many women struggle with urinary or fecal incontinence. Pelvic floor dysfunction can go on to become pelvic organ prolapse (POP), which affects the ability to get pregnant in the future. POP happens when the walls of the vagina begin to fall, and the pelvic organs (bladder, rectum, and uterus) fall with it. Sometimes it's just pressure in the vagina or rectum, or a visible bulge into or out of the vagina. And it's not always urinary or fecal incontinence — sometimes it's the opposite and urination or bowel movements are difficult. For women, the pelvic floor affects sexual function including libido, vaginal lubrication, sexual arousal, orgasm, and overall sexual satisfaction. If your pelvic floor muscles are weak, strengthening them with Kegels (rhymes with bagels) can improve your desire to have sex. Attempting to conceive for most couples means a lot of sex, and frequent sex can lead to pelvic floor discomfort. If things become too painful, it may deter your desire or ability to continue. If you have painful vaginal sex, using a fertility friendly lubricant and learning to relax your pelvic floor is very important — Kegels will not be helpful. Instead, focusing on pelvic floor lengthening while belly breathing and a few yoga poses like happy baby, deep Malasana squats, and figure-four pose can help. If you have a condition like endometriosis, painful intercourse may also be related to increased odds of infertility and should be addressed by a doctor.

Pelvic floor dysfunction doesn't just happen to women. Weight-lifting, cycling, and dropping testosterone levels can cause it in men too. In men, a weak or tight pelvic floor can lead to erectile dysfunction like less-firm erections and premature ejaculation. If you have a tight and weak pelvic floor you may need to learn how to relax its muscles with the help of a pelvic floor therapist. If the pelvic floor is just weak, Kegels can help to strengthen it.

How to Kegel

Many people think the core Kegel movement has something to do with squeezing your butt. This is not correct. A proper Kegel utilizes the same muscles you use to stop a stream of pee. Doing that a few times next time you're in the loo is the easiest way to know that you are using the right muscle group—just stop peeing, hold that feeling for three seconds, then release again. But please, don't do this regularly, as pelvic floor exercise while peeing can send mixed signals to the brain and instigate pelvic floor dysfunction. While you should not clench your butt cheeks together, there should be an anal squeeze like you are trying to keep back gas. Kegel basics are the same for men and women, though the thought exercise is different.

Kegels for women: While seated with a straight back, think about sitting on a marble and gently lifting it into your vagina. Start with a three-second pull in, then release for three seconds. Some women also imagine it as drawing a tampon into your body, then releasing it.

Kegels for men: Men can find their pelvic floor muscles through the stop-peeing trick or by tightening the muscles that help keep them from releasing gas. Start with the same stop-the-pee stream for three seconds, release for three seconds, and repeat. Following the same cues, you can also channel your inner elephant and try lifting your penis like a trunk.

Lengthening the pelvic floor

For a muscle to function correctly, it must not only be strong but flexible. If you find yourself having difficulty squeezing, it might be because your muscles are weak, or they are so tight you simply don't have the range of motion to squeeze any more. This can make vaginal penetration difficult. To lengthen the pelvic floor, try lying on your back with a pillow under your knees. Inhale deeply, allowing air to fill your low belly and all the way down into your pelvic floor. Allow your pelvic floor to relax and lengthen down, away from your trunk. On exhale, return your pelvic floor to its resting or neutral position. Repeat this for several breath cycles until you feel the gentle release of your pelvic floor muscles.

If you are experiencing reduced desire or discomfort with sex that's limiting your ability to conceive, or your partner is experiencing ED or you are unsure if your pelvic floor is functioning correctly, seek professional help. There are physical therapists who handle all issues and training and retraining of the pelvic floor. Insurance generally covers their services, so check your benefits. You can use the Academy of Pelvic Health Physical Therapy website (www.aptapelvichealth.org) to find one near you. A physical exam is helpful, but if there isn't anyone close by, therapists are available via telemedicine too.

Exercise Wrap-Up

- Moderate exercise of all kinds is great for fertility. Even a quick walk!

- Too much intense exercise has negative impacts on male and female fertility.

- Sorry, men—if you're thinking about conception, drop your cycling habit.

- Activity should feel sustainable—try to choose something you can stick to over the long term.

- Ensure your pelvic floor muscles are functioning to prepare your body for pregnancy and bonus: improve your sex life.

Chapter 9

CHEMICALS, DRUGS, AND THE ENVIRONMENT

How everyday products and the world around us
shape our fertility—and the health of future children

Saturnism was the name the Romans bestowed upon lead poisoning, an unfortunate condition caused by exposure to lead in water pipes, makeup, and amulets that decreased men's sexual function and reproductive abilities. Between the 1930s and 1960s, a form of synthetic estrogen known as diethylstilbestrol (DES) was prescribed to more than five million women to prevent miscarriages and premature births. While rodent studies showed it to be carcinogenic, it showed no serious health effects in humans. However, the children of the women who took it were another story. DES daughters had a higher risk of rare cervical and vaginal cancers, abnormalities in their reproductive organs, and ectopic pregnancies, and more than 40 percent were unable to achieve a full-term live birth. DES sons experienced reproductive abnormalities like undescended testicles, smaller-than-normal penis size, and noncancerous growths on their testicles. As recently as the 1950s, anxious pregnant women were prescribed a cigarette or glass of wine to soothe their nerves. Now we know that alcohol and nicotine are teratogens, or substances that cause abnormal physical development and birth defects during pregnancy, especially in the first trimester. Recreational drugs, alcohol, tobacco, chemicals, some viruses and bacteria, and uncontrolled health conditions like diabetes are all teratogens. These negative lifestyle exposures can also transcend pregnancy. For example, the children of parents in professions that expose them to chemicals and dust are more likely to develop allergies. House painting during pregnancy, even while putting together a nursery, puts babies at risk for eczema.

Genetic changes alter your body's DNA sequence. But the way genetic traits are expressed, meaning whether a gene is turned on or off, is influenced by behavior, lifestyle, age, and environment. Imagine your genome, your body's complete set of genetic material, as a string of twinkly Christmas lights and each light is a single gene. Epigenetic markers can turn each individual light on or off. These changes start before you vacate the womb, and are fluid throughout your life, so based on your lifestyle and exposures, your epigenome will look different as a sixty-year-old than it did as a baby. Epigenetic marks can be inherited or accumulated over time, meaning that some changes can be passed on to children and their children and their children's children. Not all epigenetic changes are negative, and unlike genetic changes, many are reversible. But smoking, for example, can cause multiple markers to change both in future children and in the woman who smoked while pregnant. Chemicals found in cigarette smoke, like arsenic and formaldehyde (yes, really—please stop smoking), can damage and break DNA, and when new strands are synthesized, they aren't always repaired properly. Your body's inability to metabolize and break down carcinogens is what can lead to different types of cancers. While the word *epigenesis* has been around since 1650, the term and ideology around *epigenetics* was only defined in 1942, and scientists still debate whether the environment truly influences the epigenome or, if it does, exactly how that process works.

We are in a perilous moment as a species. The hazardous chemicals present in our daily lives and climate change do not favor human health or reproduction. Scientists are only beginning to understand these impacts, so we don't even know what we don't know. In the United States, skin care and cosmetic products labeled as "natural" or "organic" are often anything but. Pharmaceuticals are the only products reviewed with true rigor by the FDA, which means that, like supplements, problems are found only after they occur, and labeling does not always reflect what is inside. Retailers that demand ingredient transparency are often the last line of defense against unsafe products that would otherwise hit shelves. Environmental chemicals, like those found in manufacturing and agriculture, are not subject to comprehensive testing regarding their long-term effects or impacts on human reproduction either. And no products or chemicals are tested as safe for fetal development due to the ethical concerns involved in running those studies. Human activity, like the burning of fossil fuels like coal and oil, is contributing to another fertility killer: climate change. An increasing number of wildfires are polluting the air we breathe and hurting our overall health too. The heating of the earth has effects on male fertility (sperm hates heat) and may hurt women's as well. And just like climate change, scientists believe chemical pollution now exceeds our "planetary boundary" or the limits of earth's ability to recover from human effects on natural processes.

A large and famous literature review suggested that exposure to chemicals is the primary cause of fertility and sexual-development issues for both genders. Sperm counts and quality have gone down, and girls began entering puberty earlier in the past fifty years. Miscarriage rates are rising along with the prevalence of other fertility issues. And these changes are not just happening in humans. Dog semen quality has dropped, and genital anomalies like increased intersex ambiguity have been observed in reptiles and mammals. The growth of these problems maps directly to the dramatic increase in exposure to natural and synthetic chemicals in the past several

decades; seven hundred new industrial chemicals are now introduced to the market each year. Our only conversations on this topic
today center around avoiding exposure to teratogens during pregnancy, but chemical and environmental exposures of all kinds are
vital to avoid during the preconception period too. These exposures
affect fertility in several ways: endocrine disruption, damage to the
male and female reproductive systems, and their potential to impair
the viability of a fetus.

Beyond the changes we experience as individuals, the concept
of prenatal programming explains how our bodies before and during pregnancy influence the development of our future children.
Fragmentation of the DNA inside sperm, caused by lifestyle and environmental factors, is a cause of recurrent miscarriage. Teratogenic
agents like prescriptions, nicotine, and alcohol have the greatest likelihood of impacting an embryo's development between fourteen and
sixty days postimplantation—before many women know they are pregnant. Fetal exposure to smoke, for example, can manifest later as decreased genomic stability, heightened risk of mutation, altered brain
development, clinical depression, and metabolic stress. A father's
nicotine use can lead to cognitive problems and ADHD in their children, and eventual grandchildren, via epigenetic changes to sperm.
A mother's marijuana use can affect her fetus's brain development
in utero too. Increasing prenatal phthalate exposure is causing male
babies to be born with smaller penises. Economists found that fetal
circumstances negatively impact test scores, educational attainment,
and income too.

It's impossible to avoid everything as microplastics are raining from
the sky. And as we were told as schoolchildren, we are what we eat,
and microplastics are now present in over half of human feces. Take a
deep breath, and after reading what follows, direct your energy at what
you can control, hard prepregnancy nos like smoking and drugs, and
eliminating as many teratogenic and endocrine-disrupting products as
you can at home or in your workplace.

AN OVERVIEW OF ENDOCRINE-DISRUPTING CHEMICALS

Endocrine-disrupting chemicals (EDC) mimic natural hormones in the body, fooling it into thinking it should overrespond (i.e., inflammation) or do so at an inappropriate time. Found mostly in household and personal-care products, they can do everything from stimulating the production of insulin when it isn't needed to triggering changes to the composition of intestinal microbiota. EDCs can also block hormones from functioning properly or cause over- or underproduction, like an over- or underactive thyroid. One example of how endocrine disruption directly hurts fertility is by creating a loss of blood sugar control, which can cascade into conditions like type 2 diabetes and metabolic syndrome. One-third of men who have type 2 diabetes go on to suffer from hypogonadism, or low sex drive, as the testes cannot produce enough sex hormones. Endocrine disruption can significantly impact women with PCOS, worsening the risk of lower overall fertility and gestational diabetes, hypertension, and preeclampsia during pregnancy. To jump start your household purge, here is an overview of the most egregious endocrine-disrupting offenders and where they are found.

Plastics

It's hard to buy any foods, even lettuce or tomatoes, that are not packaged in plastic. While plastics serve roles as stabilizers, dyes, colorants, UV inhibitors, and flame retardants, they are also found inside of foods, especially fish, as they feed on the overwhelming amount of plastic waste in the ocean. A recent study identified plasticizers hiding in a variety of fast foods too, including hamburgers, fries, chicken nuggets, burritos, and cheese pizza, due to the gloves fast food workers wear and plastic delivery containers. Interestingly, the levels were higher in burritos than hamburgers, and cheese pizza was most immune from contamination. Exposure to diisononyl phthalate (DINP), a phthalate that makes plastic more pliable, causes cancer

and birth defects and rains down hell on normal hormonal functioning. And now, in addition to feces, microplastic pollution has
been found in the bloodstream. One study showed its presence in 80
percent of otherwise healthy volunteers. Microplastics break down
due to temperature, water, air, mechanical abrasion, and UV light.
During pregnancy, microplastics have been detected in the placenta,
which serves as the only source of oxygen and nutrients for a growing
fetus and starts to form during implantation before a pregnancy is
even detectable.

Bisphenol A (BPA)

A well-known endocrine disrupter called BPA is used to manufacture
water bottles and food containers and print thermal receipts. It can
linger in the body for a week or more just from a dermal exposure.
In women it's known to negatively affect puberty, ovulation, and can
result in infertility, and cause chromosomally abnormal eggs and
embryos, leading to increased miscarriage rates. In men, it is linked
to changes in motility, morphology, and DNA damage in sperm. And
for both sexes, it is associated with diabetes, obesity, cardiovascular
disease, thyroid dysfunction, developmental disorders, and cancer.

Parabens

Parabens, common preservatives in cosmetics, foods, and pharmaceuticals, are easily absorbed into the human body, where they act
like estrogen. Their presence is linked to breast cancer and congenital disabilities. While the EU has safety limits to the concentration of
parabens allowed in consumer products, the United States does not.
If you're looking at your shampoo ingredients, you'll find it at the
end of a long chemical name like propylparaben or isobutyl paraben.
They can also decrease sperm production dramatically along with
testosterone levels. In animal tests, researchers observed reduced
anogenital distance and tinier testicles in offspring exposed to parabens during pregnancy. While they can bioaccumulate in the body

and live in fat tissue, levels in urine can drop as much as 45 percent after stopping exposure for three days.

Pesticides

Whether it's a topical treatment, collar, or spray, while managing your pet's fleas and ticks you are inadvertently exposed to registered pesticides. Many of these products contain ingredients that are unsafe for children or pregnant women, like the organophosphates and carbamates found in flea treatments. If gardening is your passion, wear gloves when handling pesticides or herbicides and choose green products whenever possible. Exposure to pesticides like dicamba, glyphosate, and organophosphates decrease fertility overall, and when used in large amounts on fruits and vegetables, men's sperm count drops by half and normal morphology by a third. Living near or working in the agricultural industry is fraught for male fertility and tied to developmental abnormalities like undescended testicles or abnormal urethral formation in the sons of fathers in that profession. Women who are exposed to pesticides containing a chemical called trans-Nonachlor were three times more likely to develop endometriosis. Polychlorinated biphenyls (PCBs) are oily liquids or solids with no smell or taste used in industrial contexts that also negatively impact fertility, so if you work in manufacturing, check to see if any exist in your workplace. Women with high levels of exposure to PCBs have a 50 percent decrease in ability to get pregnant, are more likely to miscarry, and less likely to achieve pregnancy when undergoing IVF. The higher the levels of PCBs, hexachlorocyclohexane, and dichlorodiphenyltrichloroethane (DDT) found in the blood, the lower a woman's overall fertility.

AVOIDING ENDOCRINE-DISRUPTING CHEMICALS

Ob-gyns are encouraged to advise their patients of exposure risks during preconception appointments, but this guidance is not a standard of care. Rarely is it given outside of that context or ever to men. Unless you're working in a chemical manufacturing warehouse or in farming with exposure to significant volumes of pesticides, it's unlikely that any physician is going to go into detail about your environmental exposures. Since most people do not book a preconception appointment, nor could all of this be covered in the fifteen minutes spent with a physician anyway, it's best to take control of these exposures yourself. Any time (like right now) is the right time to take stock, even if having children is years off.

To help you avoid their multisyllabic terror, here is a handy chart showing where the most common EDCs are found. A few macro tips: eat organic fruits, vegetables, and meat as often as possible (as many of the worst offenders are ingredients in pesticides); be picky about your seafood, since they can't be organically fed and harvested; and clean out products in your house that contain these ingredients. Skin care ingredients like retinoids and salicylic acid are important to eliminate as they trigger changing hormone levels and are known to cause birth defects during pregnancy—even in those early weeks when you may not know you are pregnant.

Personal-Care Products

Ingredient	What is it?	Labeled as
Aluminum chloride hexahydrate	Common ingredient in high-powered antiperspirants	Aluminum chloride hexahydrate
Chemical sunscreens	Sunscreens that create a chemical reaction and work by changing UV rays into heat, then release that heat from the skin	Avobenzone, homosalate, octisalate, octocrylene, oxybenzone, octinoxate, menthyl anthranilate, and dihydroxyacetone

Ingredient	What is it?	Labeled as
Formaldehyde	A known carcinogen found in personal-care products, including hair-straightening treatments, nail polish, and eyelash glue	Formaldehyde, quaternium-15, dimethyl-dimethyl (DMDM), hydantoin, imidazolidinyl urea, diazolidinyl urea, sodium hydroxymethylglycinate, and 2-bromo-2-nitropropane-1,3-diol (bronopol)
Hydroquinone	A skin-lightening agent used to treat conditions such as chloasma and melasma	Hydroquinone, idrochinone, and quinol/1-4 dihydroxy benzene/1-4 hydroxy benzene
Parabens	A common preservative in cosmetics used for its antibacterial and fungicidal properties	Propyl, butyl, isopropyl, isobutyl, and methylparaben
Phthalates	Chemicals added to plastics to make them more flexible (plasticizers) and to increase the strength and effectiveness of or dissolve other ⇨	BzBP, DBP, DEP, DMP, or diethyl, dibutyl, or benzyl butyl phthalate

Ingredient	What is it?	Labeled as
Phthalates (*cont.*)	chemicals; found in perfume, nail polish, soaps, body washes, shampoos, and cosmetics but also in vinyl flooring and lubricating oils	
Retinoids	Ingredient in prescription acne and antiaging medications	Retinoic acid, retinyl palmitate, retinaldehyde, adapalene, tretinoin, tazarotene, and isotretinoin
Salicylic acid	Acne, exfoliating products (like combination peels), and cleansers	Salicylic acid
Triclosan and triclocarban	A chemical that helps prevent the growth of bacteria and fungi	Most used as an ingredient in toothpaste, deodorants, soaps, and liquid hand and body washes; can also appear in cleaning products

Food and Physical Products

Ingredient	What is it?	Labeled as
Bisphenol A (BPA)	Chemical used in production of polycarbonate plastics like eyewear, water bottles, epoxy resins that coat metal food cans, bottle tops, and water supply pipes as well as thermal receipts	Most plastic products have a number label that can tell you whether it contains BPA. The tell is inclusion of the numbers 3, 6, and 7 inside of the recycling symbol. Items with 1, 2, 4, and 5 generally do not contain BPA.
Flame retardants	Chemicals applied directly to fabrics or other materials to prevent the start or slow the growth of fire, including furniture and seat covers (foam, upholstery, mattresses, curtains, and carpets); electronics, including computers and household appliances; electrical wires and cables; clothing; and car seats	Upholstered furniture with foam inserts made before 2015 often contains it, but it's possible to swap out the inserts with cleaner materials. Anything made after that date must have a tag stating that flame retardants are present in the material. The same is true of car seats.

Ingredient	What is it?	Labeled as
Pesticides and herbicides	Used to kill unwanted organisms in crops, gardens, public areas, and parasites in medicine; most exposures to pesticides and herbicides happen though diet or environmental exposure	Unless it's a product you purchase for use in your garden, there aren't labels when these materials are used in public spaces, nor are there warning labels on foods identifying the products used to grow them. If you're a gardener, buy green products like botanical pesticides (pyrethrum and limonene), microbial or biological agents (microbes, parasites), and inorganic minerals (boric acid, limestone, and diatomaceous earth), and avoid glyphosate. Buy organic fruits and vegetables whenever possible.

BEHAVIORS THAT HURT FERTILITY AND FUTURE PREGNANCIES

Smoking

This one is simple: smoking in any of its forms—cigarettes, cigars, vaping, chewing, e-cigarettes, or cigarillos—is harmful to male and female fertility overall and even worse during pregnancy. Exposure to secondhand smoke is harmful too. If it's hard to quit, start the process long before you choose to conceive.

Recreational drugs

Do you really need me to say it? Recreational drugs are not good for your fertility. Cocaine, opiates, meth, cannabis (see next section for more), and most others seriously affect male and female fertility and, with enough use, cause permanent damage to the reproductive organs.

Cannabis

There is a perception that because it is derived from a plant (as is cocaine, by the way) and because it is legal in many places that cannabis is completely safe. Cannabis is nuanced. Tetrahydrocannabinol (THC), the plant that marijuana comes from, and hemp, the power behind most cannabidiol (CBD) products, are two different types of cannabis plants. They are nearly identical compounds, but THC gets you high, and CBD does not. While medical marijuana is used to reduce symptoms related to cancer treatment, Alzheimer's, epilepsy, glaucoma, and multiple sclerosis, the pharmacological effects of THC on fertility are uniformly negative for men and women but especially to sperm. If you're a man who loves THC-powered products, stop using them at least three months before you try to conceive.

CBD is now found in just about everything, from oils and tinctures to stress-relieving sodas and snacks, and because it's so ubiquitous, most people believe it's 100 percent safe. More research is required, but unfortunately what we know to date does not support that assumption, and some products are not labeled clearly with warnings for those TTC or already pregnant. CBD's known fertility-related side effects include decreased sperm count, depression, fatigue, weight gain, and abnormal menstrual cycles. The other big problem: some products labeled as CBD actually contain THC. CBD was first extracted from the cannabis plant in 1940, and comes in three different extract types: isolate, full-spectrum, and broad-spectrum. Isolate is a highly processed form of CBD, full-spectrum is a blend of all eighty-plus cannabinoids from the hemp plant (including less than 0.3 percent THC), and broad-spectrum is a blend minus even small amounts of THC. The most common varietal found in sleep, sex, and relaxation aids is broad-spectrum as the combination of all cannabinoid types creates a synergy called the entourage effect that amplifies the therapeutic benefits and reduces side effects. The safest thing to do considering it's not a particularly well-regulated industry yet is to avoid any cannabis products while trying to conceive and pregnant unless you're under a physician's care.

Injectables

If you are contemplating what happens to your Botox or filler habit before you conceive, the answer from your dermatologist or injector will probably be better safe than sorry. No one really knows how injectables affect pregnancy or fertility because the research has not been performed. The only data we have is from a survey of twelve physicians funded by Allergan, the manufacturer of Botox, and it did not draw any resounding conclusions. Another review of the impacts on pregnancy over a twenty-year period did not show any meaningful impacts either. For men we know even less, as tiny studies done in animals show conflicting data and good luck gathering enough men who will admit that they get Botox. If you talk to an ob-gyn their answer will be no to all injectables simply because we don't know for sure, and in most cases it is not a medically necessary treatment. Botox can be used for overactive urinary bladder problems, migraines, and dystonia, and if taking it is a medical necessity, use is up to your doctor. If you want to be cautious, get work done three months prior to TTC.

Avoiding vaccines

Because this is still the subject of so much misinformation—especially related to the COVID-19 vaccine—it bears mentioning that even though it's been debunked repeatedly, remaining unvaccinated is far worse for your fertility. The mRNA vaccines developed to combat COVID-19 do not sterilize men, nor is there any link to infertility for either sex. The opposite is true in this case: unvaccinated men encounter transient fertility issues after they are infected with COVID-19. Women reported disruptions to their menstrual cycles postvaccination, and taking the data from almost four thousand women, there was a less-than-one-day increase in menstrual cycle length, but there were no changes in the length of a period. And there is further nuance that applies to any infection or immune response and the menstrual cycle. During the luteal phase, between ovulation and your period, your immune system is suppressed, we think to prevent your body from rejecting a potential embryo as it tries to implant. So your body's ability to fight off or manage anything new, from a virus or chronic condition to a vaccine, is diminished during that time regardless, which can cause an irregular menstrual cycle. There is no proof that traditional vaccines derived from the diseases they protect against hurt fertility either, and women should get up to date on vaccinations before conceiving.

CLIMATE CHANGE

Wildfires. Air pollution. Floods. Species-level extinctions. Rising sea levels and floods. Climate change is caused by increasing levels of greenhouse gases from burning fossil fuels, livestock, industry emissions, and vehicle exhaust that get trapped in earth's atmosphere.

Poor and vulnerable populations are impacted disproportionately, as extreme weather and natural disasters cause geographic displacement, food insecurity, exposure to toxic substances, and water contamination, as well as vector-borne illnesses like West Nile, dengue, Lyme disease, and malaria. The aftereffects can cause mental health conditions like depression, anxiety, and PTSD.

Heat in some parts of the world is now at the maximum of human's ability to survive, with temperatures over 122 degrees Fahrenheit in Pakistan and India. At some point, humans will not be able to evaporate off the heat, and massive deaths are expected, first in the global south. And it may not be that far off for the rest of the world. For the first time, in the summer of 2021, Canada experienced a heat wave with temperatures up to 115 degrees Fahrenheit that caused many deaths from heat exhaustion. The way we're headed, these temperatures will be considered cool by future generations.

Heat

The effects of heat on pregnancy are well documented. Each additional degree above eighty degrees Fahrenheit decreases the birth rate, possibly since heat reduces sexual activity. Heat also increases the rate of birth defects, especially during the first trimester, and may lead to more miscarriages. Many studies conclude that excess heat also reduces birth weight, especially in areas with generally cooler climates, as well as increased maternal hypertensive disease and placental abruption. Heat affects the ability to conceive, as evidence suggests egg and sperm are sensitive to thermal stress.

Sperm are particularly at risk with rising temperatures (a peril of external genitalia) as spermatogenesis requires low temperatures. Temperature can also change the motion pattern of sperm, which is correlated to its ability to fertilize an egg. Women's ovaries and other reproductive organs are protected deep inside of the body and shielded from these changes, but at some point, if temperatures continue to climb, they will be affected too.

Air pollution

More than 3 percent of all premature births in the United States are attributable to air pollution, and it kills more than ten million people globally per year. Air pollution has a negative impact on male and female fertility, from altering the quantity of sperm and quality of eggs to impacts on their genetics and epigenetics. Living near major roadways can cause infertility and living next to oil refineries or fossil fuel production plants causes preterm birth (as does fracking) and contributes to fertility issues. The groups that are affected most by these factors are the least likely and financially able to access fertility treatments and healthcare—low-income, disadvantaged populations that live or work in machine or industrial jobs. There is an association between preterm birth and particulate or sulfur-based air pollution. Maternal exposure to air pollution is correlated with childhood obesity and higher BMI overall in children later in life too.

Wildfires

Ob-gyns are starting to caution patients who live in areas that are especially susceptible to wildfires not to conceive during that season, or if they become pregnant, to leave to avoid exposure to airborne particulate matter and unhealthy air. But 92 percent of the world now lives in areas where the level of fine particles in the air, smaller than 2.5 micrometers in diameter, exceeds the minimum safety standards set by the World Health Organization (WHO), and is usually a direct result of car exhaust, factory emissions, wildfires, and woodburning stoves.

Raging wildfires, especially in the American West, have become common. The timing now transcends typical fire seasons and happens during the winter, a season that traditionally did not allow for uncontrolled burns. The increasing exposure to smoke and the tiny nanoparticles you can't see also negatively affect fertility. Female firefighters are twice as likely to miscarry as the general population and are more likely to experience preterm births. Self-reported miscarriage was two times more common in that population than female nurses, who experience similar stress and chemical exposure. Male firefighters are 50 percent more likely to seek fertility treatments than the rest of the population.

Birth strikers

The other effect climate change is having on fertility is forcing people to face a decision about whether to have children at all. Birth strikers list climate change as one of the top reasons for not becoming parents. Fifty-eight percent of people in one poll stated they were reconsidering having more or any children because they were concerned about the world their kids would inherit. One in four said they were considering adoption instead of biological children. A third of those asked plan to move to a different geographic area and have fewer babies thanks to climate change. Another poll showed that more than 96 percent of people were concerned about their current or future children's well-being in a climate-changed world.

Since climate change has an outsize impact on world economies, and economic factors affect fertility, fertility patterns in general are changing. It's driving some men and women to go even further and pursue sterilization—climate vasectomies or tubal ligations—in their twenties. In the past, physicians would have been reluctant to perform these procedures, given that studies demonstrate higher rates of regret at that age. But recently, doctors are taking a more patient-centered approach to conversations about permanent sterilization, as complete bodily autonomy means directing your reproductive life, including the choice not to have children.

TAKING BROAD ACTION

If you've read this far you probably wonder what you can do to mitigate any of this other than living in a cave or donning a tin hat and respirator. Here are a few major commitments to consider if you are passionate about these issues: Drive an electric vehicle (EV) or commit to making the car you own your last gas-powered vehicle. Switch to a clean-energy plan powered by solar and wind if your utility provides it or add solar to your home. Cut consumption of animal products, especially those derived from our bovine friends, cows and sheep, who emit an order of magnitude more methane than other farm animals.

On a policy level, push leaders—from the mayor to the CEO of your company and members of Congress—to put more climate-friendly policies into practice. The biggest impacts come when we focus on the gigatons, or the Big Five greenhouse gas emitters, as well as reducing major greenhouse gases themselves—CO_2, fluorinated gases, methane, and nitrous oxide. Supporting organizations that help guarantee girls education and access to birth control so they control how and when they start families will take global CO_2 emissions down by gigatons per year too.

On an individual level, be more methodical when it comes to the products you choose. If you are planning to conceive and it's an option (even temporarily), choose a geography that is less apt to natural disasters like wildfires and extreme heat, and a profession that does not expose you to toxic chemicals. Transitioning to a mostly plant-based diet free of the antibiotics, chemicals, and plastics found in animals is another tangible change that can help your body (remember 80/20 is great!). And if you want to take things to the next level, there are environmental doulas and fertility coaches who can purge problematic products from your life and tests you can buy that will measure your exposure to different substances.

Chemicals, Drugs, and the Environment Wrap-Up

- Look for EDCs listed on the labels of your personal-care, home-cleaning, and gardening products—even if they are labeled as "natural" or "organic."

- Avoid eating, drinking, storing, or microwaving food in plastic containers.

- Don't drink water from soft plastic water bottles (reusable stainless is great).

- Eat organic fruits and vegetables (and support local farms!).

- Ensure fish is from a high-quality source and eat less bovine-derived (beef especially) meat.

- Cook in stainless steel or cast-iron pans instead of nonstick cookware.

- Try steaming clothes instead of dry cleaning.

- Remove your shoes before entering your home.

- Watch the air-quality index (AQI) and limit outdoor activities and close windows on days when it is high.

- Buy an indoor air filter if you live in an area prone to wildfires.

- Avoid high-traffic areas while exercising.

I'll say the quiet part out loud: the use of these fertility-harming chemicals will not stop unless we demand it. Their release into nature is causing phenomena like algal blooms, which are growing rapidly around the world, and they release toxins that make humans sick. Impacts vary based on species and geography and are mostly presented by companies and regulators in the context of lost sea life, but if it's killing animal and plant life en masse, it's hard to imagine there are no harmful effects on us too.

Chapter 10

MENTAL HEALTH

How to manage when you're TTC
or in the throes of an infertility journey

We'll skip recounting the antics of Freud and Jung and get right to it. Enduring five pregnancies and giving birth somewhat traumatically to two now very frisky boys was the most transformative and stressful period of my life. I used grief counseling to process the first two miscarriages so I could relax somewhat before our first son was born, as I was an anxious mess looking for anything and everything to go wrong. During my season of infertility, I also had to learn how to be happy for others but sad for myself. I wasn't always good at it. During an outing with a pregnant friend, I had to leave early to go home and cry. Seeing her cute bump and glowing happiness was too much. I felt despair and primal anger for what had happened to me and envy in my bones. And I was happy for her. But I was devastated for myself.

Not everyone encounters these issues—hopefully you won't. But even if conception is smooth, you will face challenges to your mental health while pregnant or parenting, which is why learning the tools that help you cope now is so important.

So here is a reminder that it's okay to be sad. It's okay to have moments where you are in fact not happy for your pregnant or new parent friend and perhaps even resentful. All feelings are valid feelings. Work through them in whatever way works best and try to make peace with the reality that you are not fully in control of this process. That was, for me, the hardest thing to reconcile, that even with good behavior and habits and choices, things do not always work out the way you want, when you want.

I've tried pretty much everything in this chapter to cope and am still a work in progress. But the number one way I reset even now is a warm soak in Epsom salts with a book before bedtime. My other mental health salvation is the opposite—moving my body, mostly chucking heavy things, and running around listening to loud rock music.

Mental health and fertility are indelibly connected, and infertility, like every other disease, is nuanced and multifactorial. Dealing with it is rarely as simple as getting a massage, having sex, and getting a positive test. If you run into a delay getting pregnant, someone will suggest that you "just relax and it will happen!" *Shakes head* If you hear this from a well-intentioned friend or family member, remember they mean well and shake it off, or ask for a hug. A short embrace was shown to reduce women's cortisol levels, but hugs do not work the same way for men.

While the more familiar parts of fertility management we've discussed—food, exercise, and supplements—are all important, the brain brings it together. The brain affects every aspect of our health and provides the master set of instructions for our body to function, which includes firing hormones. The hormone that most negatively impacts fertility is cortisol. It is the body's primary stress hormone, and you can think of it as an alarm system that controls your moods and fear levels. It helps your body deal with stress and replenishes its energy supply. Elevated cortisol levels can lead to weight gain, make weight loss harder, and weaken your immune system if elevated for too long.

The complex system of feedback loops and pathways that control the secretion of cortisol is called the hypothalamic-pituitary-adrenal (HPA) axis. The HPA springs into action after it is triggered by negative feedback loops, which can be as subtle as feeling anxious or worried, or bigger emotions like fear or trauma. When the HPA receives these signals, it releases cortisol and norepinephrine, which tell your liver to break down and release glucose. When there is a big enough trigger, the HPA kicks the body into fight-or-flight mode to conserve energy, sometimes making it temporarily insulin-resistant. To counter this reaction, simple techniques like diaphragmatic breathing and meditation can bring the HPA back in balance. Mindfulness exercises lower the risk of developing metabolic syndrome in individuals struggling with depression. Pertinent to fertility, the HPA mediates stressors via metabolism, immune response, and the autonomic nervous system. Once you're pregnant, neonatal exposure to repeated stress responses can reprogram a baby's brain, shaping the way their HPA axis later functions as an adult.

Cortisol flares related to practical aspects of baby-making like finances, work, mental transitions, and conception can cause suppressed LH secretion and disrupted ovulation. Women with higher levels of alpha-amylase, an enzyme that indicates stress, are 29 percent less likely to get pregnant. Cortisol has an inverse relationship with sperm production and reduces motility and concentration for men. Increased levels make sugar cravings more acute and slow metabolism, leading to weight gain. Women who experienced one or more stressors in an hour burned 104 fewer calories, which is equal to almost eleven pounds of weight gain per year.

Reactions to infertility can be very different. Women more frequently report depression and anxiety and respond more poorly to treatment failure. Though men experience some stress, they do not appear as emotionally affected, are less likely to seek help, and are more willing to consider terminating treatments. This disconnection often causes friction in relationships, so if you're pursuing fertility preservation or assisted reproduction, take the clinic's offer of counseling as it is tailored specifically to those experiences. They have interventions designed for everything from fertility preservation, enduring the two-week wait, and even helping men overcome their fears and prepare for a semen analysis.

Mental health problems are common, difficult to diagnose, interconnected with the rest of our lives, and can be transient so they are often pushed aside. But they shouldn't be. You and everyone else you know will at some point struggle with stress, anxiety, depression, or something more serious. Triggers can range from lingering childhood trauma, life changes, the daily hits of cortisol while reading the faster-than-ever news cycles, or the less expected causes like allergies, which are associated with a 66 percent increased risk of psychiatric disorders, 43 percent higher risk of anxiety disorders, and 38 percent risk of eating disorders. Anything you haven't resolved from childhood tends to come up when you become a parent, so process whatever you can with whatever methodology works best for you before you start that journey.

COMMON MENTAL HEALTH CONDITIONS THAT AFFECT FERTILITY

Cortisol spikes are a trigger for hormone changes, which can go on to cause fertility issues. The mental health conditions these spikes cause vary in severity and while some are transient and acute, others stick around for a while. While stress alone does not cause infertility, side effects like low sex drive can impair the ability to get pregnant.

Stress and anxiety

More than 70 percent of adults report feeling anxious or stressed every day. Stress manifests differently for everyone but is defined as feeling overwhelmed or unable to cope with emotional or physical adversity. Acute stress is short-term, and usually happens after a stressful event. It decreases the body's resistance to infection and impairs the ability to mount a strong immune response, and yes, it impacts your fertility too. Chronic stress is long-term and can last months or even years. It causes insomnia, fatigue, low sex drive, appetite changes, weight gain, difficulty concentrating, and impairs T-cell immunity, which can put the body at risk of tumors.

Anxiety is the most common mental health condition in the United States, and the main drivers include brain chemistry, environmental factors, and genetics. Anxiety is rooted in our will to survive, and often is not about the situation we find ourselves in but instead the way that we think about what's happening. Symptoms range from feelings of dread or fear, rapid heartbeat, feeling restless, wound-up, or easily fatigued and irritable. When acute, it can manifest as an anxiety attack and includes symptoms like feeling dizzy or faint, dry mouth, excessive sweating, and restlessness.

Dealing with regret is a universal aspect of dealing with infertility that causes stress. Whether it's wishing you'd started TTC sooner or blaming yourself for a miscarriage (please don't!) we have all been there. Here is a short list of my infertility regret and how I've come to accept my experience: why didn't I try to have kids earlier (couldn't find the right partner), these miscarriages mean there is something seriously wrong with me (nope, likely just an aging egg supply), my eggs are scrambled because I had an extra glass of wine at dinner (just meiotic errors, which again, are due to age), the placental issues I had while pregnant with my second son were because my uterus sucks (this may be partially true, though more likely caused by complications from two D&Cs and a prior C-section than born that way). I'll stop there, but my point is, no matter what happens, there is usually an answer that points to biology, not a choice you made or anything you can control.

Depression

Anxiety creates feelings of worry or dread, and while those can be aspects of depression and the conditions often coexist, depression is characterized as feeling hopeless, sad, and living in a low-energy state. Because its symptoms vary and are self-reported, depression is difficult to diagnose. Symptoms of major depression include increased or decreased appetite, lack of energy and interest in activities you usually enjoy, feelings of worthlessness or guilt, trouble concentrating, and in more extreme cases, suicidal thoughts. You need at least five of those symptoms for more than two weeks to receive a depression diagnosis, which happens during an interview with a health provider.

Depression can be an underlying cause of erectile dysfunction or a side effect of infertility. Infertile men are 48 percent more likely to develop heart disease, 30 percent more likely to develop diabetes, and have a higher risk of abusing alcohol. Dealing with these conditions can also exacerbate depression. There is also a reciprocal link between depression and obesity, as obesity doubles the risk of depression and depression is predictive of developing obesity. For women, the link between infertility and depression is similarly pronounced, and its presence can make the underlying causes of infertility worse.

Premenstrual dysphoric disorder

Eighty percent of women experience PMS symptoms during the luteal phase of their cycle, and most resolve after their period concludes. Premenstrual dysphoric disorder (PMDD) is a more amplified version of PMS, and affects 3 to 5 percent of women. A PMS diagnosis only requires one symptom, which can be anxiety, confusion, depression, irritability, bloating, breast tenderness, headaches, or weight gain. For PMDD there must be five symptoms present in the week before your period, with improvement and eventual absence as your period starts and in the week afterward. These symptoms are mood swings, irritability, depression, feelings of hopelessness, anxiety, decreased interest in things you usually love, difficulty concentrating, fatigue, changes in appetite, insomnia or hypersomnia, feeling out of control, or any of the physical symptoms of PMS like bloating, breast tenderness, weight gain, or joint and muscle pain.

PMDD treatments alleviate physical and psychological symptoms, starting with a prescription for oral contraceptives to manage hormone imbalances. Selective serotonin reuptake inhibitors (SSRIs), the class of drugs that are used as antidepressants, are then used to treat psychological symptoms. If you run into difficulty tolerating SSRIs or birth control, the only supplement with solid evidence to help treat mood disorders is calcium. And the next topic we'll cover, cognitive behavioral therapy (CBT), is a great complement to SSRIs or as a standalone treatment too, especially if you are TTC.

THERAPY IS AWESOME

We have doctors for every body part, financial advisers, lawyers, personal trainers, and car mechanics to help manage other aspects of our lives. Our minds deserve a little love too. Therapy is helpful whether you're trying to navigate a new job, new geography, relationship issues, career questions, are on a journey of self-discovery, or, pertinent to this discussion, thinking about or actively TTC or experiencing infertility. Seeking help doesn't mean you are weak. Humans are social creatures, and we were never meant to deal with so much alone. If you plan to become a parent, buckle up—that little adventure is *all* about knowing when to ask for help.

Medications can help balance body and brain chemistry and trim off the highs and lows, but the most common way to treat mild or moderate anxiety is cognitive behavioral therapy (CBT). It provides the tools to let go of unhealthy thoughts and process past experiences.

A very simple example: not many people like going to the dentist. The negative feelings that develop over time can prevent you from going at all when they aren't dealt with. And this behavior can spread to other areas of your life, interfering with other areas of medical care. CBT helps you identify your anxiety triggers and disrupt the stress spirals so you can cope in the moment.

Therapy is still mostly a one-on-one relationship with a provider unless you're doing it with a partner or friend. If chatting from your couch is more appealing than trekking to an office, telemedicine allows access to mental health providers via video, voice, or text. Meditation and mindfulness apps are here for asynchronous support or to self-manage. Apps and VR offer asynchronous escape and mindfulness programs on-demand to abate stress solo. And cohort-based, expert-led programs with others in the trenches provide community and social support. Many of these programs come with the option to get a prescription for a variety of drugs. But before you begin taking any medications or antidepressants, discuss if or how all medications could impact your fertility or future pregnancy. Some medications prescribed to help support mental health are fertility-friendly and many are not, so it's essential that you review carefully. If it's a heavyweight prescription, see someone for a second opinion before filling it.

The goal of therapy is to break a habit, not mitigate its effects. The real work happens when you address your inner fears or unspoken needs, deal with unresolved trauma or family issues, or take on a struggle with anxiety or depression. CBT helps to work through negative thought patterns or behaviors to prevent them from happening again. Its practices are designed to help you change the way you think and then change the way you feel about or act during certain situations. Digital CBT programs are prescribed for everything from treatment of irritable bowel disorder to erectile dysfunction. Touted as side-effect-free, their outcomes are as good and, in some cases, better than prescription drugs.

MENTAL HEALTH MEDICATIONS AND THEIR FERTILITY IMPACTS

From categories like selective serotonin reuptake inhibitors (SSRIs), serotonin and norepinephrine reuptake inhibitors (SNRIs), atypical antidepressants, tricyclic antidepressants, or monoamine oxidase inhibitors, the impact of mental health medications on fertility varies from zero to serious. Although many people have positive outcomes, around one-third of the nine million adults in the United States treated for depression also find out theirs is treatment-resistant and does not respond to any drugs. Medicating PTSD sufferers is even less promising with today's options. And even if they work, many are not appropriate to use during pregnancy or while trying to conceive.

For men, SSRI use is linked to fertility issues including lower sperm count, decreased motility, higher DNA fragmentation, decreased libido, ejaculation problems, and erectile dysfunction. If the SSRI is responsible for these changes, they can be reversed given three months' time off it. For women, SSRI use causes similar issues with sexual function like low libido, but does not appear to affect ovarian function, egg quality, hormone levels, or negatively impact outcomes during IVF treatments. Fertility aside, taking SSRIs during pregnancy is not advisable unless there is no alternative, since they are linked to increased risks of miscarriage, birth defects, preterm birth, newborn behavioral syndrome, and neurobehavioral effects later in life. Continuing an SSRI during pregnancy should be a decision between you and your care team, weighing the risks and benefits.

CBD is used by an increasing number of people who don't want to use medications to manage their mental health. And it works for insomnia, can increase libido, reduce anxiety, stop seizures and chronic pain, and eases depression. But a reminder from the previous chapter that we don't know a lot about its effects on fertility. Until we understand more about its long-term effects, stop using any cannabis products three months in advance of trying to conceive so egg and sperm production are free of possible side effects.

Stopping medications abruptly leads to its own set of issues, and SSRIs can make symptoms worse or cause new ones to appear. If you do need to stop, tapering is ideal. With that in mind, talk to your prescribing physician about other options six months or, if possible, a year in advance of trying to conceive. Making a medication change can be hard, and it can take time to taper down or off if necessary, and sometimes it involves tweaking the dose or trying several before you find one that works. If you are using CBD or any other herbal medications, you should also talk to your physician about conception and pregnancy-safe alternatives so you or your partner are not left managing the emotional, sometimes anxiety-inducing first trimester with no assistance.

OTHER WAYS TO WORK ON YOUR MENTAL HEALTH

Acupuncture

You might be wondering why acupuncture is in the mental health chapter. Though it has many benefits, one that nearly everyone who tries it cites is a feeling of deep relaxation during and after treatments. Acupuncture is the most frequently suggested complementary practice during fertility treatments and for improved overall fertility, so much so that some fertility clinics employ an acupuncturist in-house. Acupuncture has been used in China for more than twenty-five hundred years, as an analgesic for chronic pain and a single anesthetic technique for surgeries as serious as craniotomies and open-heart procedures. A literature review of fifty-six studies concluded that craniotomies that combined general anesthesia with acupuncture led to faster extubating and postoperative patient recovery, reduced nausea and vomiting, and potentially protected brain tissue. Its inability to fit into the construct of Western medicine means that medical school doesn't teach it, it's not performed in a traditional doctor's office, and the clinical studies that do exist are rarely published in well-respected, mainstream medical journals. Caveats aside, at a minimum, pretty much everyone can benefit from a soothing chat followed by a forced nap.

Appointments start with a brief medical and lifestyle history to talk about concerns and any problems you'd like to address. They'll look at the color and shape of your tongue, and the strength of your pulse, then insert tiny needles the width of a hair into specific points on what Chinese medicine considers to be the body's vital energy, called qi. The precise placements into the central nervous highway system of qi, or meridians, stimulates and releases endorphins, serotonin, dopamine, and other hormones that make you feel good. Don't be surprised if needles do not go directly into the areas that you are targeting—that isn't how acupuncture works. For stress and anxiety, popular points are the top of the head, between the eyebrows (the third eye for any yoginis), shoulder well, chest center, and points in the hands and feet. The needles are very thin, and there is no pain or discomfort when they are inserted, just a slight ache if they hit a sensitive area.

Other practices that can make appearances are forms of acupressure and massage, gua sha (using a stone tool to scrape the skin to relieve pain and tension), cupping (using heated cups that act like vacuums to improve blood and lymph circulation), and Chinese herbs to support your overall health. If you decide to take herbs, ensure you coordinate them with your other providers, as there can be interactions with medications.

Licensed acupuncturists (their names are followed by the acronym LAc) must attend school for an average of three to four years culminating in the completion of a master's or doctorate, then pass an exam, perform at least one thousand clinical hours, and meet licensure requirements that differ by state. Look for a practice that focuses specifically on fertility or women's health, and if you need a referral, ask friends, your ob-gyn, or reproductive endocrinologist.

Mindfulness

Mindfulness is a catch-all description of practices that help us be more present, creating awareness of what we are doing and where we are, and it helps us avoid being overly reactive day-to-day. It is a tool to help us observe and understand our thoughts and feelings and sensations in our bodies, a talent most people lack in today's digital, always-on world. Mindfulness practices come in many forms, from breathwork to meditation and even aromatherapy, and they can have huge impacts on conditions like depression. Compared to standard mental healthcare, mindfulness-based cognitive therapy is even effective in preventing relapse in recovered depression patients. Its major benefits during a fertility journey are the ability to better cope with stress and anxiety, which drives down cortisol levels, and to provide the tools to better process and be present during the experience.

Breathwork

Distilled to its essence, breathwork retrains your body to breathe more deeply. Techniques range from belly breathing to resonant breathing and lion's breath (which you may have encountered in yoga class), and popular options are available in books, online courses, or a guided app. If you want to try it out, the five-five breath, or coherent breathing, is a good daily option to slow down anxious moments. The goal is to breathe more deeply at a rate of five times per minute. Start the exercise by paying attention to your natural breath cadence to see how long your inhales and exhales are. Then move into a deep inhale for four seconds, and exhale for four seconds for one minute. In your next minute, move to a five-second inhale, then exhale and step your way up to ten seconds for each over time. This practice can start at five minutes per session, and gradually increase to twenty minutes as your practice progresses. On each inhale, visualize the stressful thoughts and feelings, and when you exhale, release them out of your body. Breathwork is a wonderful daily practice even when you're feeling good or it can defuse stressful moments. Like mindfulness, its main fertility benefit is helping regulate cortisol levels and overall stress.

Meditation

A consistent meditation practice changes the brain's structure and function. MRI scans of frequent meditators show that it activates the areas involved in problem-solving, adaptive behavior, and self-awareness, and improves memory, focus, and emotional regulation while reducing anxiety, fear, and stress. Though most of our thoughts play on repeat, and the majority of those are negative, the brain is surprisingly good at rewiring itself. Meditation helps reset the brain's thought playlist so you can get out of those unhealthy patterns and start listening to something else. It can also create physical changes, like lower blood pressure and blood sugar, and help with your immune function and sleep quality.

Yes, it's easy to fire up an app or start a program, try it once, and decide you suck at meditation. I get it. (No, really, I've done this many times). Flushing your mind of active, busy thoughts long enough to go into a trancelike state takes practice, just like anything else. Meditation is not a skill most people are born good at, and like breathwork, there are many different methodologies and tricks that help people find their zen place. Some people create a special corner of their house with a cushion and candle, others can do it anywhere if they're wearing headphones. While most meditation practices involve sitting, others suggest lying on your back à la Savasana at the end of yoga class. Eyes open or shut is up to you—whatever helps you focus. Like breathwork, it takes time to work up to longer periods of meditation.

To try meditation, go to a place that feels calm and peaceful to you with five minutes of uninterrupted time to focus. Find a comfortable position on a chair or the floor (cross-legged is fine). Then be still and pay attention to what's going on in your body. Feel your breath flow in and out, and try to slow it down. Be in your breath and try to notice your thoughts. If they wander away, don't get mad or frustrated—just bring them back and focus on your breath. Reducing your stress level is one benefit, and that reduces cortisol levels, but another is that meditation also increases your attention span.

Aromatherapy

Essential oils like lavender help relieve anxiety and promote relaxation and sleep. Aromatherapy is touted during childbirth as a nonmedical way to manage anxiety, and is also a tool to regulate stress. To try aromatherapy, you can inhale essential oils directly or add them to a bath or take it up a notch and buy a diffuser to keep in your home office or bedroom. Buy high-quality versions either from your acupuncturist or a naturopathic shop with a good reputation.

Exercise

Even though you just read a whole chapter on this topic, here it is one more time. Exercise reduces inflammation via several processes (inflammation generally, cytokines, toll-like receptors, adipose tissue, and via the vagal tone) that can contribute to better health outcomes in those suffering from mood disorders. And yes, exercise also causes the release of endorphins. Any type of physical activity you choose (practiced in moderation) has mood and fertility boosting benefits for your body and mind.

Stop drinking and smoking

Alcohol is a natural sedative, hence the popularity of nightcaps. But alcohol messes up your sleep and your balance of neurotransmitters, leading to increased levels of anxiety. A systematic review of studies on reduced alcohol consumption showed that cutting back lowers the rates and levels of anxiety and depression, among many other positive fertility-boosting effects. Smoking can be a crutch during stressful times, but the consequences are like alcohol: nicotine and other chemicals in cigarette smoke can alter your brain's pathways and make anxiety worse.

Cut down on caffeine

A fun and delicious cure for fatigue, sadly too much caffeine can make you jittery and nervous, which is not helpful if you're experiencing anxiety. Caffeine works by blocking adenosine, a neurotransmitter that helps you feel tired, and by releasing more adrenaline. So, for the sake of your fertility (and your mind), trim it down to less than two hundred milligrams per day, which is a generous sixteen-ounce pour of your favorite coffee.

Eat a healthy diet and reduce late night snacking

See chapter 6 for fertility-improving pro tips and a template to follow. But TL;DR vacillating blood sugar levels, unhealthy food, and midnight trips to the kitchen all interfere with your sleep.

Sleep!

Humans are supposed to spend around one-third of their lives sleeping, but a full one-third of adults get less than six hours of sleep per night instead of the seven to eight that is universally recommended. Getting enough sleep is associated with improved cognitive health; lower stress levels; a reduced risk of diabetes, heart disease, stroke, and obesity; and a reduction in food cravings for highly processed, caloric, sweet foods. These conditions and factors also impact fertility.

It isn't always easy to fall or stay asleep, especially if you've skimmed this chapter and identify with symptoms of anxiety or depression, two of the most common sleep disruptors. But there are simple ways to improve your sleep hygiene. Your bed is for sleeping, not for TV watching, work, or late-night snacking, and ideally your bedroom is dark and cool. Going to bed and waking up at a different time every day throws off your body's clock, so try to find a schedule that works and stick to it.

A consistent wind-down routine is another way to train your body to sleep on schedule. If you struggle with relaxing before bed, try a warm bath, or a breathing or mindfulness exercise. Other sleep pro tips include not eating giant meals, and not using nicotine products, or taking caffeine within a few hours of bedtime. Caffeine should be avoided at least four hours before you plan to go to sleep. Exercise is great for sleep, but night workouts can wake your body up, so try to get your steps or activity in at least ninety minutes and preferably three hours before bedtime. If you really can't sleep, don't lie there, or toss and turn for hours. Get up and go to another room and read a book or whatever makes you feel calm so you can reset and try again.

Forest bathing

Even if you live in a city, walking outside surrounded by trees benefits everyone. Meandering even briefly through a forest, or forest bathing, has physiological and psychosocial effects, inducing relaxation and stress reduction. Negative feelings like anxiety, depression, anger, hostility, confusion, and fatigue all get lower. On a macro level, city dwellers, in general, are more stressed out and have an increased risk of health problems, especially mental health disorders. They are on more medications for mental health issues as well, so it's especially important to occasionally escape the concrete jungle and get outside to a park or, better yet, the wilderness.

Soak up some sunshine

If you've experienced jet lag, you know how messing with your sleep-wake cycles can influence everything from your appetite to your mood. Humans are solar-powered creatures, and like Superman we rely on exposure to sunlight to function properly. Our retinas have photoreceptors that react to particles of sunlight and trigger the brain to run genetic, hormonal, and neurotransmission processes that affect the activity of the brain and most other cells in the body. Erratic

sleep and not enough sun exposure throws off these processes, causing weight gain, acne, depression, and gut issues.

Our sleep-wake cycles have an official name: circadian rhythms.
Managed by your body's circadian clock, it regulates almost all systems in the body in some way, and when the rhythm is off, cognitive
impairment, psychiatric illness, metabolic syndrome, and cancer can
follow in varying degrees. Its main cue is daylight, which turns genes
that control its molecular structure on and off. Exposure to sunlight is
linked to the neurotransmitter serotonin, which modulates our moods,
and a decrease can cause mood disorders, from increases in anxiety to
seasonal affective disorder, which can manifest as major depression.
Our skin may help to produce and regulate serotonin too. But it is why
seasonal changes tend to bring on changes in our moods.

The field of chronobiology seeks to understand the natural biological rhythms related to solar and lunar cycles. Off-kilter biological clocks have been tied to common chronic health conditions like
obesity, diabetes, depression, bipolar disorder, and sleep disorders. A
better understanding of biological clocks could help treat jet lag, mental health disorders, and obesity, and help workers adjust to nighttime
shifts. Pertinent here, when our circadian rhythms are off, our stress-
response system is too. Though research is still early, we know that our
clock genes influence our stress hormones.

Try starting the day with a little direct sunshine and see if it changes
your mood or health. At bedtime, avoid artificial and blue light to signal to your body that it's time to go to sleep. Yes, that means a stop to
your screen time.

Mental Health Wrap-Up

- The hormone that most negatively impacts fertility is cortisol, the body's primary stress hormone.

- Cortisol is triggered by negative feedback loops in the HPA axis, which can be as subtle as feeling anxious or worried, or bigger emotions like fear or trauma.

- There is no "right" way to manage your mental health, and what works for your friends, family, and partner may not work for you.

- Options range from therapy, meditation, exercise, and acupuncture, or can be as simple as getting outside for a walk.

- Feeling stress and anxiety from time to time is a normal part of starting a family. If you are navigating a fertility challenge, most clinics offer therapy tailored to that experience.

- If you've had suicidal thoughts, please speak to someone you trust and seek professional help. If you need immediate assistance, The Suicide and Crisis Lifeline is available twenty-four hours a day, seven days a week by dialing 988.

- Asking for help doesn't make you weak; it makes you human.

Part 3

Taking Action

Chapter 11

MAKING BABIES

The ins and outs of getting pregnant

The specifics of human reproduction were hotly debated for centuries, as it calls into question religious beliefs and cultural practices. Aristotle fathered the theory of epigenesis, or the idea that life spontaneously generated from materials found in the egg. His writings went on to inspire the preformationists, who believed humans developed from tiny versions of themselves held in sex cells. But it wasn't until 1760 when a priest put frogs in taffeta pants that we started to truly understand how things worked. An Italian physiologist named Lazzaro Spallanzani realized that the wormlike creatures in semen were important, but not exactly why. He also believed that physical barriers could play a role in allowing (or not) pregnancy and turned to amphibians for proof. In what can only be described as an unfortunate and embarrassing situation for male frogs, he dressed them in tight-fitting pants and let them loose in a tank of females. None of the females became pregnant, as the pants acted as contraception. A century later, Louis Pasteur closed the book on spontaneous generation. He boiled meat broth in a flask with a long, swanlike neck that allowed the free flow of air but not dust particles. The broths were bacteria-free unless the flask was broken open, which proved that, in Pasteur's words, "life only comes from life."

We know now that humans exist thanks to autonomous generation, and while a cell develops spontaneously it requires both male and female gametes to make an embryo. Who a person becomes—how they look and their predisposition to certain traits—is contained in their DNA. Nearly all complex organisms on planet Earth reproduce this way, with very few exceptions. Several insect and animal species like bullhead sharks can reproduce asexually or alternate between sexual and asexual reproduction, an ability known as heterogamy. Humans, not so much.

Human reproduction is a beautiful, complicated dance of signals and cells that must work together perfectly to create life. At the beginning of each menstrual cycle, the pituitary gland releases follicle-stimulating hormone (FSH) to trigger the maturation of a few eggs in each ovary. As the largest dominant follicle grows, estrogen levels rise to inhibit the secretion of FSH, signaling the nondominant follicles to die off. When estrogen is high enough, luteinizing hormone (LH) is released to trigger the final stage of egg maturation, ovulation, and the collapse of the nest-like follicle after the egg escapes. That collapsed follicle transforms into the corpus luteum. It releases progesterone, signaling the other follicles not to release further eggs, to tell the uterus to build up its lining, and to change the quality of cervical mucus, the cervical position, and basal body temperature (BBT).

The egg then journeys through a fallopian tube toward the uterus. If it encounters sperm on this trip it is fertilized, and the combination of cells continues its week-long trip toward the uterus. An intense period of cellular division along the way converts the fertilized egg into a blastocyst, the stage at which the embryo can implant in the now lush uterine lining. When it does, human chorionic gonadotropin (HCG) is released to remind the uterus not to shed that thick lining. The presence of HCG in urine is what causes that second line on a pregnancy test to turn pink as it rarely appears in the body for any reason other than pregnancy (though some tumors produce it, and your thyroid can mimic it).

The corpus luteum continues to release progesterone for eleven more weeks until the placenta is ready to assume its duties maintaining the endometrium and nourishing the fetus. And bam! It's a pregnancy.

Okay, so have sex, sperm meets egg, mission accomplished, right? Well, getting pregnant even with a standard penis-in-vagina scenario isn't always that simple. A lot of what happens after you have sex is completely out of your control, and if you get pregnant once, the experience can be very different every subsequent time. Regardless, everyone has questions. Like is doggy-style or missionary more effective? Do women have to orgasm to deliver the sperm to the egg? Should I lay on my back with my feet in the air afterward? If so, for how long? The truth of optimizing sex for procreation is more boring than you want it to be, and the short answer to those questions is, although gravity and deeper penetration deliver sperm closer to their destination, there is no one method or position to rule them all.

A question that doesn't come up as often as it should: How do I keep things interesting if we've been trying for a while? Timing sex can start to feel like a job and finding the perfect moment for both of you to get in the mood may prove impossible after a few months. It also turns out, just like fertility, trends in sex are on the downswing. The number of young men reporting no sexual activity—alone or with a partner—rose from 29 percent to 44 percent between 2009 and 2018. For women, it jumped from 50 percent to 74 percent during the same period. Rough sex behaviors like choking are more common now too. Yikes. Years of being marooned in the same spaces during the pandemic haven't helped. But we don't really know why our relationship with sex is changing. It could be partly to do with changing gender norms or exposure to porn and photoshopped bodies or because women are challenging structural misogyny in their work and personal lives. So, if you find yourself looking at the less than spontaneous sexual component of conception with some trepidation, you aren't the only one. Talk to your partner about timed sex and any other issues before you get started. And if you encounter baby-making fatigue, there are solutions. At-home ICI (intracervical insemination—please don't use a turkey baster, there are FDA-cleared kits!) is a solution that many couples now turn to, especially if it's taking a while. It's also a worthwhile option before pursuing IUI or IVF if there are certain types of ejaculation issues in play.

BEFORE YOU GET PREGNANT

Beyond stopping birth control with enough time for your fertility to return to normal and monitoring your cycles for any irregularity or new symptoms, book a preconception appointment. Yes, male partners—this means you too. What you cover in a preconception appointment depends on the practitioner. Women should prepare for a Pap smear and breast exam, blood tests for STIs, get up to date on vaccines, especially those that cannot be administered during pregnancy, examine all medications they are taking, eliminate those that can cause harm to a pregnancy, and add medications, like insulin or thyroid meds, if diabetes or thyroid disease are a concern. There is a connection between periodontal disease, like tooth decay and gum disease, and poor pregnancy outcomes, so book an appointment with your dentist too (and don't skip the flossing). Most ob-gyns only take appointments when you're already pregnant, though there can be exceptions, so this will likely happen with your gynecologist. (Fun fact: just like all toads are frogs but not all frogs are toads, all ob-gyns are gynecologists but not all gynecologists are ob-gyns. The latter takes specialized training.)

Men should expect a similar routine with a physical exam done by a primary care provider. First appointments do not include hormone testing or semen analysis unless it's indicated. In addition to answering your questions, they'll have a few for you, like how many kids you'd like to have, a current list of prescriptions, and (as you'll do many times throughout this process) a full medical, surgical, and family history. They'll also dig into your lifestyle and much of what we've discussed in previous chapters.

PRECONCEPTION APPOINTMENT CHECKLIST

Appointments for women:

☐ Gynecologist visit with Pap smears

☐ Breast exam

☐ Baseline laboratory tests

☐ Genetic screening and STI test (optional or if indicated)

Appointments for men:

☐ Visit with a general practitioner

☐ Genetic screening and STI test (optional or if indicated)

☐ Semen analysis (order a kit online or pick one up at the store) .

For both:

☐ Dentist for X-rays and general care

☐ Vaccine update (chickenpox, rubella, hepatitis B, measles, and mumps)

Even if you decide to skip the preconception appointment (but seriously, just go), at some point while starting a family you will work with a team of medical professionals in a meaningful way. This can be fraught—from reasons like previous experiences with medical racism, fear-related anxiety, or not enjoying the vibe of a clinic or hospital. And really who does? The physical design of most healthcare settings is terrible. As a patient it is your right to ask any questions you want, for as long as you want. Informed consent is a critical part of the relationship with every healthcare provider you encounter. Here are a few tips to become your own best advocate during that preconception appointment and beyond.

- **Prepare for your appointment:** Bring a list of questions along with your symptoms and any other general concerns so you don't forget anything.

- **Take a buddy**: You are entitled to support during an appointment. Whether it's a partner or friend, this person can be your notetaker, or just hold your hand during a potentially difficult conversation.
- **Access, review, and save your records**: Almost all medical practices utilize electronic medical record systems known as EMRs, so a record of your appointment and past appointments with other providers is available online any time you want to look at them. Before you leave the office, ask how to log in and export your records so you always have them.
- **Get a second opinion**: If you leave your appointment wondering if you are on the right track, consider seeing another provider for a second opinion. Before you do, ensure your insurance will cover it or else you risk paying out of pocket. However, in some cases, especially if the procedure is invasive or expensive (and nearly all of them are) it is worth the extra money to be certain you're doing the best thing.

HOW TO GET PREGNANT FAQ

**You wrote a pregnancy book,
so do you have a get-pregnant-fast playbook?**

Sure do! Track your ovulation for at least three months prior to TTC using whatever method is your favorite (basal body temperature monitoring, cervical mucus method, fertility sensor, peeing on an ovulation tracking stick, or a combination of several for the most accurate results). Pinpointing that fertile window is everything. Women, stop douching (preferably permanently), cut back on alcohol, stop using all drugs (including all forms of cannabis), and check your lubricants to ensure they are sperm-friendly. Men, if you haven't stopped using the sauna, hot tub, or other places that heat your testicles, now is the time. Same with cycling.

Both of you should drop your exercise intensity down to moderate. Five days before ovulation is set to occur, have sex every other day including the day of ovulation. Sperm can live for up to five days in the female reproductive tract, and frequent ejaculation lowers sperm count and can increase the percentage of immature sperm, reducing the odds of fertilization, so sex once per day is the absolute max. For good luck, ladies stay on your back for ten minutes afterward to let gravity assist. Then fill your life with distraction during the two-week wait (TWW) and take a pregnancy test first thing the morning after your period is late.

Wait, why shouldn't I just have sex on the day I ovulate?

An egg survives only twelve to twenty-four hours after its release, so you may miss your window if you time your only shot with the basal temperature spike. If you're using an OPK, tracking BBT, or see that egg white–like cervical fluid, you should time an attempt with that LH rise. Having sex in the days before ovulation (once per day or every other day is plenty) maximizes your chances since sperm is so resilient. If your partner has a low sperm count, he should abstain from ejaculation for a few days before your fertile window to build up a good supply.

Can I time sex to optimize for a boy or a girl?

Methods like Shettles and Whelan are very light on evidence (read: unproven). So the short answer is although it can be a fun way to keep things interesting, there is no proof that any have bearing on the gender of a future child.

What can I do and not do during the TWW?

The dreaded TWW can feel like the two-year wait. For those not familiar with fertility parlance, TWW is the time it takes for a pregnancy test to show (or not show) that second line thanks to the presence of human chorionic gonadotropin (HCG). So, will a glass of wine during the TWW cause a miscarriage? Can you have that extra cup of coffee? The best and safest way to approach the TWW is to treat it as if you are pregnant. Keep your consumption of alcohol to a single glass of wine or beer, or preferably cut it altogether. No drugs including cannabis. Caffeine is fine in moderation, meaning a medium-size cup of coffee or tea each day. The best activity is staying distracted to keep your mind off the what-ifs (and if-nots).

When can I take a pregnancy test and get an accurate result?

Wait until a missed period and do it first thing in the morning, as HCG levels are highest before you dilute your urine with morning coffee or other liquids. With today's more advanced tests, you can start peeing on sticks up to five days before a missed period if you are cycle tracking. If you have PCOS or your cycle is irregular, it's harder to predict. Delayed implantation can cause a false negative since HCG levels are too low for tests to detect.

Different tests come with specific instructions and timing for an accurate result, and they can also go bad if not stored correctly or for too long, so follow directions carefully. False negatives aside, chemical pregnancies, or very early miscarriages, are another reason to wait to test. They are thought to happen in 50 to 60 percent of all first-time pregnancies and show the same HCG surge. They can be caused by low hormone levels, inadequate uterine lining, or an infection, but most of the time are due to chromosomal abnormalities. Unless you test early, you won't even know it happened.

What are early signs I might be pregnant?

Early pregnancy signs feel like PMS, so overinterpret at your peril. The most obvious sign is a missed period, but others include cramping, frequent night peeing, changes in tastes and smells, fatigue, implantation bleeding (spotting), moodiness, nausea, and sensitive nipples. Implantation bleeding can be confusing and happens to around one-third of women when the embryo implants into the uterine lining. Signs it's implantation bleeding and not your period are timing (it happens about ten days after ovulation), the duration is usually hours instead of days, discharge color is a lighter pink or brown versus a period's cranberry red, and cramping is milder than PMS without growing intensity.

Any nonobvious pro tips for early pregnancy?

If congratulations are in order, you can level up and read my first book, *Bumpin'*, which is packed with all the tricks to manage pregnancy. But here is something I wish every pregnant woman knew in those first weeks. Avoid infection. It sounds obvious, and who likes being sick, but the first trimester is when there is the most risk of problems with fetal development. A pregnant woman's body is in an immunosuppressed state so that the growing baby isn't rejected or attacked since it is technically an outside organism. If the mother's immune system is overstimulated, it can go after the embryo or fetus, causing problems ranging from birth defects to mental disorders. Infection also puts pregnant women at risk for preeclampsia, premature delivery, and miscarriage. So don't hang out with sick people, wash your hands for at least twenty seconds, and try not to touch your face too often. Keep up with your flu and COVID-19 vaccines—they have no adverse effects on pregnancy, whereas getting either will make you miserable and can cause serious complications. Skip raw and undercooked foods (especially meat), and wash vegetables thoroughly too. If you have a partner, ensure they follow the same rules.

How long does it take for the average couple to get pregnant?

Healthy couples in their twenties have a 25 to 30 percent chance of getting pregnant during each menstrual cycle, and 84 percent of all couples who TTC are pregnant within one year. The qualifier is that they must be off contraception and have regular sex, which is defined as every two to three days. Age also plays a role. For women between nineteen and twenty-six years old, 92 percent will conceive after one year and 98 percent will in two years. It slowly declines from there, and between ages thirty-five to thirty-nine drops to 82 percent after one year and 90 percent after two years. After forty, the per-cycle odds of getting pregnant go down to one in ten.

It's been a while and we still aren't pregnant. When should we seek help?

The guideline for couples under thirty-five (more specifically when the female partner is under thirty-five) is to seek professional help after twelve months of trying with no luck. For couples over thirty-five, it drops to six months. If you have medical conditions or other factors that make it more complicated to get pregnant, seek care when you feel you need it, which can be earlier than this guidance or before you ever start. However, most providers stick to these rules before they refer out to a reproductive endocrinologist.

PARTNER MEETING

Welcoming a baby is life-changing and amazing and not always easy. If you have a partner, things will change. A lot. There will be exhaustion and fights and moments where you don't like each other much. It passes—when you talk about it. These questions are designed to proactively address the most common issues couples tackle from conception through newborn life. Find a quiet time, answer honestly, and you'll head off these problems before they start.

1. Describe your life in five to ten years. How far away from this vision are you now?

2. Where do we want to live? City or suburbs, near family, schools, etc.?

3. Why do you want children?

4. What about your childhood did you love? What wasn't great?

5. What did your parents do well, and how did they disappoint?

6. How many children do you want? Would you prefer a boy or a girl? Why?

7. Which aspects of starting a family are you most excited about? What scares you?

8. Do you want to pursue preconception testing like genetic or carrier screenings? What would you do if the results revealed bad news?

9. How do you feel about assisted reproduction treatments like IVF?

10. How do you think your relationship will change after having a baby?

11. What is most important to you as a couple—quality or quantity time?

12. How do you plan to carve out individual time so you can maintain separate friendships and hobbies?

13. How do you manage stress, and what kind of support do you need if you're navigating something difficult?

14. Who is your parenting role model? Why?

15. When it comes to co-parenting, which aspects do you look forward to the most? The least?

16. How do you plan to divide household labor and childcare?

17. How does each of you plan to navigate returning to work? Will both of you return to work?
18. Do you have childcare preferences like day care, a nanny, or family help?
19. Who is your backup if something happens to one or both of you (guardians, wills, etc.)?
20. How much are you willing to spend to have a baby? Who will maintain the budget?
21. Are there any cultural traditions you'd like to incorporate into family life?

Making Babies Wrap-Up

When	What to Do
Between one year and six months preconception	Schedule a preconception appointment. Assess the products in your home and swap out as needed. If you are on medications that are not fertility-friendly, make an appointment to find a substitute. Start to build sustainable activity and dietary habits that you can stick to over the long term.
Three months preconception	**Women:** Start taking prenatal vitamins, double-check all personal-care products. If you still aren't getting a regular period, set another appointment with your ob-gyn or gynecologist. Track your cycle and ovulation to find your fertile window. **Men:** Supplement if needed (or just take a multivitamin), check exposures, stop cycling, avoid hot places (saunas, hot tubs, computers in the lap, etc.) that will hurt your sperm production. **Both:** Eat healthily. Find ways to relax and keep your cortisol levels down. Talk about how you're feeling. Stop any recreational drugs.
One-month preconception	Ratchet down your activity levels if you haven't done so already to moderate levels. Relax!

When	What to Do
Actively TTC	Keep your alcohol levels low or stop altogether. Ensure your lubricants are fertility-friendly. Check in if things feel stressful or if you are struggling. Asking for help does not make you weak!

When most people decide to get pregnant, they prefer that it happen as quickly as possible. As someone who got pregnant four out of five times on the first shot, I can tell you the single most important piece of data is when you ovulate. Also, my conception genes are strong—my mom and grandmother had no problems getting pregnant. But beyond ovulation and fertile relatives, I treated the preconception period like most people do the months before their wedding, taking time to connect to my body and improve my lifestyle. So did Nick. Because unlike a wedding where the main benefit is nice photos and fitting into a big white dress, the reward here is a healthier pregnancy and healthier future children.

Chapter 12

FERTILITY TESTING

Finding answers whether you are fertility-curious or struggling to conceive

One of the first known female fertility tests was touted in the fourth century's Hippocratic corpus: inserting a head of garlic into the vagina for the night, then trying to smell it through the mouth the following day. Whether it was a misshapen uterus, misaligned cervix, or out-of-balance humors, there were treatment suggestions galore for women: vaginal fumigation, inflating the uterus and filling it with cucumber, or consuming inhuman amounts of garlic until flatulence occurred. No tests or treatments were included for men. By the mid-nineteenth century, an Italian neurologist and physiologist named Paolo Mantegazza correlated semen characteristics with male fertility. He suggested that semen volume was the main indicator, a big leap since male infertility assessment was relegated to identifying anatomical defects at that time. With the advent of more powerful microscopes, scientists realized that sperm was more complicated than it originally appeared. In 1902, a group of researchers studying azoospermic men first suggested that a semen analysis take place before a woman is treated for infertility. And yet today, in 25 percent of infertility investigations men are not examined.

Primary infertility is defined as the inability to achieve pregnancy after one year of regular, unprotected, heterosexual intercourse. The guidelines on seeking help exist because half of couples who try to conceive for six months regardless of age will be pregnant by a year, so the battery of expensive testing and treatment before then is often unnecessary. The American Society for Reproductive Medicine makes treatment exceptions for women who have irregular cycles, conditions like endometriosis, or a predisposition to diminished ovarian reserve, and for men who have known or suspected subfertility or sexual dysfunction.

Infertility doesn't just strike prospective parents. Complications from a previous pregnancy and other factors can impact the ability to conceive in the future, a condition known as secondary infertility. Reasons range from increasing post-pregnancy age or weight, lifestyle factors like picking up smoking or drinking too much alcohol, or physical damage done to your fallopian tubes or uterus. Seek help, even if you've had a child previously, after one year of TTC if you're younger than thirty-five, and at the six-month mark if you're thirty-five or older.

Then there are people who have no problem conceiving but cannot stay pregnant. Miscarriage is thought to happen in as many as one in four pregnancies, if not more. The most common cause is chromosomal abnormalities that happen randomly during cell division. Rarely is a miscarriage related to lifestyle or anything you did like exercise or falling. Recurrent miscarriage is defined as two or more miscarriages, and it is rare—just 1 percent of women experience them. The standard to consider infertility care like assisted reproduction generally happens after three in a row. Most people choose to see a provider during a miscarriage to ensure it resolves (or for help if it does not on its own) or afterward to check in. Research into recurrent miscarriage is still nascent, but it's thought to be tied to DNA fragmentation in sperm.

One reason we don't completely understand why infertility

happens is we aren't gathering all of the data required to figure it out. The US Centers for Disease Control and Prevention (CDC) yearly assisted reproductive technology report, which gathers data from nearly all fertility clinics in the country, breaks female infertility down into subcategories—endometriosis, tubal factor, ovulatory dysfunction, uterine factor, and diminished ovarian reserves. If the reason for seeking care was related to a man's body, it is coded vaguely as "male-factor infertility." Categories like sperm motility, morphology, concentration, count, or volume and obstructive conditions like varicocele are not reported. If they were, we would have a more nuanced view of how male-factor infertility manifests, and how common these problems truly are.

In 2009, the World Health Organization classified infertility as a disease. This may seem like an unimportant or obvious distinction, but that label is what determines whether insurance or governments pay to treat it. It took almost a decade until the American Medical Association followed suit in 2017, but even now, fertility testing and assisted reproduction are still mostly cash-pay industries. While for diagnostic purposes it is done in a doctor's office, the soon-to-be $680-million fertility-testing market is here for the fertility curious with an assortment of screenings, mostly as hormone panels, from home or on demand at a lab. Flip back to chapter 4 for a peek at how those work.

If you find yourself facing fertility problems—as so many of us have—be honest when you seek care, even if you feel embarrassed. Twenty-three percent of people admit they lie to their doctors about their lifestyles. Half fudge the truth about smoking and exercise, and 38 percent diminish their drinking habits. And those are just the people who admit it. Most are dishonest to avoid embarrassment, but a quarter felt they wouldn't be taken seriously if they were truthful. Finding a fertility practitioner you feel comfortable with may take interviewing several. But it is worth the work so your journey is more collaborative and personal, and you feel heard.

TYPES OF FERTILITY PRACTITIONERS

Who you see for fertility care depends where you are on the journey. For women, it usually begins with the same ob-gyn or gynecologist you visit for a yearly check-in and is escalated to a reproductive endocrinologist (RE), an ob-gyn with additional training in fertility, for specialized care. For men who have a primary care provider (and many don't), a preliminary assessment can happen with them. If there are no clear answers, men are usually referred to a urologist or andrologist.

Andrologists and urologists

Women have gynecologists to handle their reproductive issues. Men have no equivalent for proactive reproductive care but do have two different -ologists to navigate infertility: andrologists and urologists. While the training is similar, urologists stick to diseases and general disorders of the urinary tract and adrenal glands. You can think of andrologists as male gynecologists who focus on the totality of a man's reproductive health, including hormones and the endocrine system, genetics, and physical conditions like erectile dysfunction and undescended testes. They also harvest sperm for IVF and IUI and perform vasectomies.

Reproductive endocrinologist

If you've received a referral from an ob-gyn, urologist, or andrologist, or need to pursue assisted reproduction treatments like IUI or IVF, the provider you'll see is a reproductive endocrinologist. Referred to as an RE, reproductive endocrinologists are ob-gyns who top off their eight years of medical school and residency with a three-year fellowship covering the nuances of the female reproductive system as it relates to fertility. And they don't just diagnose and treat infertility. Fertility-preservation treatments like egg, sperm, and embryo freezing are also done with the help of an RE, though if an intervention is needed to obtain sperm, an andrologist will also be involved. Finding an RE without a referral from a medical provider can be tricky, as many people don't discuss their treatments even with friends. Also REs generally require a referral to see patients, as there simply aren't enough of them. The Society for Assisted Reproductive Technology (SART) reports data on 90 percent of clinics and allows you to search based on outcomes as well as your geography, so their website, www.sart.org, is a great place to start. Most REs are found in cities, so if you live in a rural area, many offer virtual consultations in advance of making a long trip, but treatments will require that you be there in person.

FERTILITY TESTING FOR WOMEN

A first appointment starts with an extensive medical history covering everything that could be related to your fertility, including past issues like fibroids or cysts, infections, and a history of STDs and STIs (please be honest) along with a dive into your menstrual cycle. For a more efficient appointment, go in with data points about cycle length, features like regularity, length, and physical characteristics like color. If you do not know your family history or are worried there are health issues your parents didn't share, consider broaching the conversation with them. The questions your provider will try to answer first are:

- Are you producing an egg and ovulating each month?
- Are there any blockages in your fallopian tubes that may prevent sperm from getting to the egg?
- Is your uterus receptive and ready to carry a pregnancy free of issues like endometriosis and adenomyosis, polyps, and fibroids?

The concept of a hostile uterus sounds a little strange (and is an example of how outdated medical terminology can be), but the concept of uterine receptivity means that there are certain times the uterus will accept an embryo and other times that it will not. The exact timing can differ from person to person. By a lot. Implantation usually occurs between six and twelve days after an egg is fertilized, as the journey through the fallopian tube to the uterus is several days. With IVF, finding a uterus's unique window of opportunity is critical, especially in cases where routine embryo transfer fails. The test used to find it is the endometrial receptivity array (ERA), which is a genetic test and biopsy of the uterine lining. However, the procedure has only been studied in good prognosis patients and doesn't appear to improve pregnancy rates overall.

A fertility differential also includes eliminating common problems like issues with the cervix (inflammation due to an infection like a STI or STD, abnormal growths, or cervical incompetence, another rude medical term meaning the cervical opening widens before it should), ruling out endometriosis and PCOS, identifying dysfunctional ovulatory cycles or uterine and fallopian tube abnormalities, and less commonly, running a postcoital test. Yes, a postcoital test is what it sounds like—have sex and go into the doctor's office a few hours after for an examination to evaluate whether sperm can survive in the cervical mucus and make it to the reproductive organs. The most common diagnostic tests you will encounter during a fertility workup are below.

Day-three blood test

Done primarily to check hormone levels, specifically AMH, DHEA, estradiol, FSH, LH, prolactin, testosterone, and TSH, a simple blood test done on cycle day three helps to understand everything from current egg count to thyroid function. It's done on day three because that is when estradiol, FSH, and LH levels are the most stable. This is the same fertility assessment you can do outside of a doctor's office via a direct-to-consumer test. But reminder: going into your doctor's office with a copy of your at-home tests isn't enough for a clinical fertility assessment, and nearly all physicians will rerun tests in their own labs with their protocols. When indicated, some providers layer on tests for infectious diseases, a complete blood count (CBC), which is used to assess your overall health and detect disorders like anemia and infection, a glucose test, and screen for cystic fibrosis–carrier status.

Day-three ultrasound

When you go in for a day-three blood test you will also get a day-three transvaginal ultrasound. It is as awkward as it sounds—a dildo-like wand is inserted into the vagina to get a closer peek at your reproductive organs. It takes place during your period, so there will likely be some blood, but they are prepared for it (the wand is covered with a condom-like sheath), and the procedure is fast, usually just two or three minutes. Day-three ultrasounds are performed to measure follicle numbers and sizes, endometrial thickness, and to look for ovarian cysts or anything else that could interfere with a pregnancy or the success of an ART cycle. Another ultrasound later in the menstrual cycle is used to confirm that follicles are maturing, and that ovulation occurred. While a reproductive endocrinologist usually performs this ultrasound, sometimes an ultrasound tech will be in charge, and they cannot share much (if anything) in real time. You'll get a call afterward when your physician has reviewed the results.

Antral follicle count (AFC)

This test uses a transvaginal ultrasound specifically to count the number of immature follicles available to release an egg each cycle, and in combination with AMH levels indicates your total remaining egg supply. If between twenty and forty antral follicles are found, there is around a decade of fertile years left. If the number is five or less, your odds of getting pregnant naturally are low and perimenopause is imminent or in progress. Note that even if you have a lot of follicles, an AFC cannot determine their quality. Planning for egg freezing or IVF always includes an AFC pre-egg retrieval.

Sorry, there is no such thing as egg quality testing

While it seems like this should be a thing, remember that testing the quality of a human egg would destroy it, since eggs are a single cell. It is only possible to understand the quality of an egg when it becomes an embryo. Quick review of egg facts: egg quality is mostly driven by age, lifestyle factors like smoking, and health conditions including endometriosis, adenomyosis, and PCOS, and most problems occur in the three months of maturation pre-ovulation.

Endometrial biopsy

If your uterine lining doesn't get thick and inviting enough, the fertilized egg will not implant, or if it does, it will not survive for long. The purpose of an endometrial biopsy is to ensure that the uterine lining develops appropriately during the luteal phase of your cycle. It's not universally part of a fertility workup and is done mostly if you have heavy, long, or irregular cycles, or if an ultrasound detects thickened uterine lining, which can indicate endometrial hyperplasia and increase the risk of endometrial or uterine cancers. It can also be indicated postmenopause if you experience bleeding. The procedure starts like a Pap smear, then the cervix is cleaned and dilated, and a thin suction tool is inserted to collect a small tissue sample for biopsy. While the procedure takes fewer than five minutes, the biopsy results take a week to come back. Tissue sampled in an endometrial biopsy can be tested for many different things including endometriosis, endometrial receptivity, and uterine microflora. There can be cramping and discomfort afterward, so rest and ibuprofen or acetaminophen are suggested post-procedure.

Hysterosalpingogram (HSG)

There are a few variations on this multisyllabic procedure, but the goal is the same: to determine whether the fallopian tubes are open and working correctly. In concert with other diagnostic tests, it can also indicate whether the uterine cavity has surface lesions like fibroid tumors, polyps, or scar tissue. The fallopian tubes can be closed, diseased, have hydrosalpinx (think bloated sausage), or be inflamed thanks to conditions like pelvic inflammatory disease. Ectopic pregnancy (when an embryo accidentally implants into the fallopian tubes instead of the uterus, and is therefore not a viable pregnancy) can also damage the fallopian tubes and cause future issues if not resolved quickly and medically when it's detected.

A hysterosalpingogram is done in a radiology suite. The ob-gyn places a speculum in the vagina, then inserts a small catheter into the uterus. Radiographic images are taken for a few seconds while radio-opaque dye is injected into the uterus and out the tubes to show whether one or both are blocked. Some studies have shown increased fertility rates in the three months after this procedure, especially for couples who have unexplained infertility, as the dye flush may dislodge mucus plugs or other debris. Improvement was more pronounced for women who experienced a higher degree of pain, possibly because the fallopian tubes were indeed clogged. There are no awards for suffering, and this procedure can hurt, so ask your doctor about at-home pain-management options.

Hysteroscopy

Hysteroscopies are done to explore abnormal Pap smear results or uterine bleeding, postmenopause bleeding, miscarriage or unexplained infertility, uterine scarring, polyps, or fibroids, to take biopsies or remove endometrial lining or find and retrieve missing IUDs. After sedation, which can be general or just local to help you relax, your cervix will be dilated, liquid or gas is inserted into the uterus to improve visibility, then a camera is used to look around. If tissue samples are needed, a biopsy will be taken. If there are fibroids, those can be removed too. Risks are low and limited mostly to bleeding and cramps with a small chance of pelvic inflammatory disease. The gas can take twenty-four hours to escape, which can cause discomfort.

Many providers recommend not having sex or inserting anything else into the vagina for two weeks after a hysteroscopy.

Laparoscopy

Typically reserved for diagnosis or treatment of endometriosis or other pelvic disease, laparoscopy is an exploratory surgery used to view the internal pelvic area, especially the surfaces of the ovaries and fallopian tubes. It begins with general anesthesia and then several small incisions are made on the abdomen, or the procedure is performed through the belly button. The abdomen is inflated with CO_2 gas so physicians can insert instruments and a camera to look for and correct uterine abnormalities, fibroids, or perform a tubal hydration. Incisions are small and closed with a stitch or two. The most uncomfortable side effects are weakness and soreness around the incisions and gas pains as the body releases the rest of the CO_2.

Saline-infusion sonohysterogram (SHG)

The shape of the uterus can impact a potential pregnancy and impede the ability to get pregnant at all. SHG is performed to evaluate a uterus's shape, the endometrial lining cavity, and reveal more information about the ovaries. Done via a combination of ultrasound and sterile fluid, it is performed when there is abnormal uterine bleeding, recurrent miscarriage, or unexplained infertility. After a menstrual cycle concludes, an ultrasound probe is placed into the vagina along with a thin catheter that goes through the cervix into the uterus and fills the uterus with sterile saline. The liquid helps to bring definition to the uterine walls and cavity, showing possible scar tissue, fibroids, polyps, or other structural abnormalities. Complications from SHG are very rare, happening less than one percent of the time, usually as a pelvic infection when there is a blockage in the fallopian tubes. This procedure is not painless and causes cramping, so it's generally recommended to take ibuprofen before and after to manage discomfort.

FERTILITY TESTING FOR MEN

While men are not subjected to ticking-clock imagery or heavy-handed headlines claiming their reproductive years are slamming to a close, fear is a reason male fertility testing is often declined. A study of young men in the Swiss military revealed that only 38 percent had sperm concentration, motility, and morphology values that met the WHO's semen reference criteria, a standardized measure of sperm health. Nearly all young Swiss men countrywide were invited to participate, yet only 5 percent chose to pursue it. Practical issues like access to clinics were cited as reasons they declined, as was discomfort at the donation process and the genital examination. But many also admitted they were not psychologically ready to learn the results.

Male fertility assessments start the same way women's do, with a personal and family history, so bring (and be honest about) your list of known issues, conditions, past surgeries, medications, and lifestyle. Male causes of infertility fall into two buckets: obstructive and nonobstructive. Obstructive is a physical blockage or structural issue somewhere in the male reproductive parts, typically the vas deferens. A physical exam will also look for varicoceles, and in some cases a testicular ultrasound will be performed to look for cysts. Nonobstructive conditions are often due to genetic, environmental, or lifestyle factors and medical treatments like chemo and radiation that impact sperm production and quality. Another cause of nonobstructive azoospermia (no sperm) includes microdeletions in the Y chromosome that encode for spermatogenesis. A preliminary fertility assessment usually starts with a semen analysis, then pending results, can include a physical exam to look for obstructive issues and blood. A karyotype, or genetic test that evaluates the size, shape, and number of your chromosomes, can also be done to detect conditions like Klinefelter's syndrome.

Varicocele evaluation

Pronounced "veh-ruh-koh-seel," varicoceles are abnormal or enlarged veins surrounding the testicles. They are the most common and correctable cause of male infertility, found in around 16 percent of all cases referred to clinics. There are multiple theories as to why varicoceles happen but no agreed upon etiology. Varicoceles are identifiable through a physical exam or ultrasound, and in between 78 and 93 percent of cases it is found on the left side. In some cases, they resolve on their own. If they are more serious and left untreated, they can cause testicular atrophy. Surgery to correct a varicocele is usually suggested if it's found in the context of an infertility exploration, and, in many cases, it corrects sperm irregularities like low count and DNA fragmentation. Embolization is an alternative to surgery and creates a tiny dam in the vein to divert blood away from the enlarged vein. Both are relatively low-risk procedures and what is right for you will depend upon specific anatomy and if there is chronic pain associated with it.

Standard semen analysis

A semen test works the way you assume, by masturbating into a cup in a private room with audio or visual stimulation, then submitting the result for testing. To produce the best sample, abstain from ejaculation for between two and seven days before your appointment. Most lubricants and saliva can impact test results, as can collecting it in a typical condom, which sometimes contains spermicide. It's also best not to test sperm health while sick, as infection impacts its parameters. The macroscopic evaluation criteria include appearance, viscosity, odor, and pH. The semen sample is also examined under a microscope and graded on five criteria:

Motility: How well sperm move (if they can't swim to the
    egg, it's a problem).
Morphology: The shape of sperm.

Count: The total number of sperm in the ejaculate.
Concentration: The ratio of sperm per milliliter of semen.
Volume: How many milliliters of semen is produced.

The reference range is wide across these parameters because most sperm have physical deformities like multiple heads or tails, corkscrew tails, or way-too-large or -small heads, which make them less competitive when it's time to race to the egg. It doesn't matter for humans if it's above a certain threshold, since most reproduction happens in monogamous relationships, and it only takes one sperm. If there are still no answers, sperm may be evaluated for DNA fragmentation. Testing male fertility can also start at home, with direct-to-consumer companies offering testosterone and hormone screenings, semen analysis, and DNA fragmentation testing. But like hormone testing, if you are undergoing a formal infertility evaluation, at-home testing will not replace in-clinic testing, and your doctor will inevitably rerun it on their own equipment, so it's best for the fertility-curious.

DNA fragmentation testing

Sperm can look fine during a semen analysis and go on to fertilize an egg, but modifications to the genetic material within can cause big problems. The DNA inside of sperm is fragile and affected by oxidative stress brought on by infection, lifestyle, environment, and age. When the DNA becomes damaged, the resulting condition is known as sperm DNA fragmentation (SDF). It is linked to recurrent miscarriage and can hurt the odds of a successful pregnancy and assisted reproduction procedures like IVF. A test known as DNA fragmentation analysis reveals these breakages and modifications in the sperm's genetic code. It works similarly to a semen analysis, as a sample is submitted to a lab. Men with a history of cancer and couples with a history of miscarriage or unexplained infertility are prime candidates for this test. It is not part of routine care yet and often isn't done until fertility treatments have failed. But since SDF is mostly caused by oxidative stress, it can be decreased by cleaning up lifestyle and diet, reducing exposure to pollutants and heat, and wearing looser-fitting underwear.

Semen analysis diagnosis quick guide

Most clinical lab results don't come with much (if any) explanation. So, if a semen assessment hits your inbox, here are the most common words you'll see if anything is considered abnormal based on the reference ranges created by the WHO.

Aspermia: No ejaculate

Asthenozoospermia: Sperm motility less than the reference value

Azoospermia: No sperm in the ejaculate

Necrozoospermia: All sperm are dead

Normozoospermia: Normal ejaculate

Oligoasthenoteratozoospermia: Sperm morphology, count, and motility less than reference value

Oligozoospermia: Sperm concentration less than the reference value

Teratozoospermia: Sperm morphology less than the reference value

TESTING FOR BOTH

Sexually transmitted diseases and infections (STDs and STIs)

Women make up around two-thirds of all new STI infections, and the impact on fertility can be big. Substance abuse, unprotected sex, and a high number of sexual partners increase the risk of getting an STI, which can then become an STD. The tricky part is that not all come with symptoms, and undetected they can lie dormant and wreck your reproductive system. This is even more common in men. Pelvic inflammatory disease (PID) is an infection commonly caused by STDs like chlamydia and gonorrhea, which can lead to tubal factor infertility and damage the ovaries. Both can also be passed on to a baby during birth and cause corneal scarring or even blindness. Herpes simplex virus (HSV) has more indirect effects—when it is active, couples must abstain from having sex. Untreated syphilis can cause infertility in men and women and cause organ damage all over the body. Though there are many different varietals, painful sex and urination, genital warts, unusual vaginal discharge, spotting between cycles, headaches, muscle aches, and fevers can all indicate an STD. For men, the connections are less clear, but some can affect sexual performance and cause erectile dysfunction.

Please, don't take your partner's word that they are "clean." Men have higher rates of asymptomatic chlamydia and test less, so they cannot possibly know for sure. You owe it to yourself, your body, and your fertility, to take STD testing seriously even if you are in a committed relationship. Showing a negative STD test on paper should be everyone's love language before sex without a condom, especially outside of monogamous relationships. You may get tested at a yearly doctor's appointment, but if you are thinking of conceiving, it's an essential part of the prep process. If you don't want to do it at a doctor's office or feel embarrassed to discuss your sexual history (as many people do), there are at-home tests that allow you to screen for the most common sexually transmitted diseases like chlamydia, gonorrhea, hepatitis C, herpes simplex virus type 2, HIV, syphilis, and trichomoniasis. Most of these conditions are easily cured when caught.

Human papillomavirus (HPV)

HPV is common—nearly all sexually active men and women get it at some point in their lives—and very misunderstood. HPV is an STD that infects epithelial cells on the oral and genital mucous membranes and the surface of the cervix and the anus. An HPV infection does not often cause fertility issues for women, especially if it was contracted in your early twenties and cleared on its own, as it does in most cases. However, it can cause skin warts and cancer, and the removal of these abnormal cells from the cervix can cause fertility problems. These procedures also change cervical mucus production and impact the overall function of the cervix. If you received the HPV vaccine, know that it does not negatively impact fertility. In fact, it is a huge plus as it prevents the development of abnormal cells on the cervix.

For men with HPV, the story is a little different. Active HPV may have a negative effect on sperm motility, and sperm containing HPV can increase the risk of early miscarriage. The topic merits far more study as there is enough clinical evidence to pay attention.

Genetic testing

If you're one of the millions who has done at-home genetic testing for reasons beyond appeasing your mother, you understand that many health conditions, from breast cancer to Alzheimer's, show up in the results. So can traits like an aversion to cilantro, ability to sing on pitch, or whether you're likely to be an Olympic sprinter. Whether you like cilantro is another matter, as the mere presence of a genetic variant doesn't mean it is active. Epigenetic changes related to lifestyle factors can cause problems and cannot be tested. But conditions that cause fertility issues that are related to your hardwired DNA have nothing to do with your lifestyle—you inherited it from your parents—and these are detectable with testing. If you've experienced recurrent pregnancy loss or have PCOS or endometriosis or primary ovarian insufficiency, for example, there may be a genetic variant at play. Azoospermic and cryptozoospermic men have gene variants on the X chromosome that are thought to be responsible for those conditions too.

There are three different types of genetic defects: single gene, polygenic, and chromosomal abnormalities.

Single-gene defects: A mutation or abnormality on a specific gene

Example: For women, the presence of fragile X (FMR1), plays a role in ovarian function. Men with cystic fibrosis gene mutations can have missing vas deferens, low sperm count, or azoospermia.

Polygenic gene defects: A combination of multiple genes or environmental effects

Example: Endometriosis, early menopause, and PCOS can all be hereditary and associated with many different genes, making them hard to diagnose through only genetic testing

Chromosomal abnormalities: Changes to the number or structure of the chromosomes carrying the DNA, usually as an extra, missing, inverted, or translocated chromosome, though these are more rare.

Example: The most well-known survivable chromosomal abnormality is Down syndrome, or trisomy 21, which is caused by an extra copy of chromosome 21. Many others are fatal and end in miscarriage or stillbirth. Testing for chromosomal abnormalities is done during pregnancy to evaluate the viability of a fetus, usually at the ten-week mark via noninvasive prenatal testing (NIPT). NIPT is done automatically for pregnant women over thirty-five, but those under thirty-five usually must pay out of pocket. When it comes to fertility, Y chromosome gene deletions are associated with azoospermia or the absence of the ducts that allow sperm to move out of the testicles, which is why genetic testing is indicated if either condition is suspected.

Genetic conditions can also have hereditary links to specific populations. Sickle cell disease is more common in those of African or Mediterranean descent and Hispanics, while Tay-Sachs and Canavan diseases are common to Ashkenazi Jews. If any of these conditions are in your family history, genetic testing should be discussed with your doctor before you conceive so you understand the risk of passing it on. These are all single-gene conditions that are easy to test. Bigger existential questions people have about genetics cannot be answered with testing, at least not yet. Questions like how much of our destinies and physical and mental attributes are we born into via our hard-coded genetics, and how much can we control? Or how much will my eventual child resemble the mash-up I did using photo filters?

WHEN THERE ARE NO ANSWERS

In some cases, results from tests are normal but infertility persists. Fifteen to thirty percent of couples are diagnosed with unexplained infertility, as testing cannot always provide definitive reasons. A lack of exact diagnosis can cause people to obsess over and then doubt test results or make them believe something is seriously wrong. Others will have one or two results that are suboptimal but do not preclude spontaneous pregnancy, yet the cause for the low values is unknown. Lower-than-average AMH and low morphology in sperm are two examples of borderline results that cause anxiety but do not always keep people from getting pregnant. Though continuing to TTC with no answers and potentially the same negative pregnancy test feels pointless, unexplained infertility is unpredictable, and sometimes people get pregnant anyway, though this is not universally the case. Personalized treatment is critical, so before pursuing invasive and expensive treatments (and all fertility treatments are), ensure all appropriate testing for both partners was performed.

My first pregnancy ended in an early miscarriage, the second in an abortion due to a fatal chromosomal abnormality, and between the births of my two sons was a missed miscarriage, when the fetus has died but the pregnancy does not resolve naturally. Even after three failed pregnancies, testing, access to the world's foremost minds on fertility, and writing two books on this topic, I still don't know why we had such a hard time. My hormone levels were normal, Nick's semen analysis was great, and other than a gut condition and my age (thirty-five to thirty-eight during this process), I was healthy. My guess without more invasive testing (which I'm not pursuing, since our family is complete, and frankly, I can't take any more medical instruments in my vagina for a while) is that our problems were due to my age.

Fertility Testing Wrap-Up

- If you are facing fertility problems—as so many of us have—be honest when you seek care, even if you feel embarrassed.

- The only types of fertility testing you can do at home are hormone panels and a semen analysis. If you visit your favorite doctor, they will look at the result but still rerun the test on their equipment.

- Care for women starts with a gynecologist, ob-gyn, or a primary care provider and progresses to a reproductive endocrinologist. Hormone tests and an ultrasound are where most providers start their exploration, but the exact testing roadmap will be personalized and based on your specific needs.

- Men usually start with their primary care doctor (if they have one) and are then referred to a urologist or andrologist pending the specific issue. The first consultation usually involves a semen analysis and physical exam.

- Never be afraid to ask questions during appointments and take notes. If you don't understand why a test is being done, dig into it with your provider, and treat the relationship like a partnership.

Chapter 13

FERTILITY PRESERVATION

The ins and outs of freezing sperm, eggs, and embryos

Just as America declared its independence in 1776, our favorite frog-fashion-expert Lazzaro Spallanzani was busy observing sperm. Under what circumstances he made this discovery is not included in his journals, but he noted that snow (and, by proxy, temperature) rendered human sperm motionless. In 1953, Dr. Jerome K. Sherman went a step further and combined his two famous innovations—the use of glycerol to preserve sperm and gradual slow cooling and thawing—to successfully fertilize an egg with frozen sperm, leading to a live birth. Though this accomplishment wasn't reported for nearly a decade, the sperm-bank industry boomed after the news went public. Eggs had a longer journey to the freezer. In 1989, Melbourne-based Dr. Debra Gook contemplated the paucity of fertility preservation options for female cancer patients and deemed it unacceptable. Though frozen eggs were used to achieve live births in the 1980s, researchers more or less gave up after that due to their fragility. Dr. Gook found a liquid that replaced some of the egg's water, allowing for them to be frozen more slowly, and went on to open the world's first egg bank. Her work paved the way for other pioneers, like Dr. Nicole Noyes and Dr. Eleonora Porcu, who used egg freezing during IVF cycles to preserve extra retrieved eggs rather than throw them out. And with the advent of vitrification, or rapid freezing, outcomes improved enough to push egg freezing out of obscurity.

Egg freezing was labeled as experimental until 2014, due to the limited data on the efficacy, cost-effectiveness, and the emotional risks. It went mainstream after this tag was removed, and many employers now offer it as a benefit.

Outside of medical need, egg freezing is positioned as a cornerstone of "having it all" and a social choice to preserve a woman's fertility until she is ready to have children—an insurance policy of sorts. This leads most women to believe egg freezing is a guarantee when really it isn't. The retrospective cohort study previously mentioned showed that the live birth rate for thawed eggs across all age groups was just 39 percent, and what mattered most was the age at which eggs were frozen; the younger, the better.

Since it is relatively new, there are still many aspects we still do not understand, like how long an egg can be frozen and later unfrozen successfully or the long-term effects of freezing on future children. Many women also assume that egg freezing is simple and noninvasive. But a single egg retrieval requires multiple trips to a fertility clinic, hormone shots taken over a series of days, an anesthetized minor surgical procedure, and high upfront costs and what can be more than a decade of storage fees. Egg freezing is essentially an IVF cycle that stops before the egg is fertilized and the embryo is transferred.

Even though sperm freezing is simpler, cheaper, less invasive, and the practice is older, it is still done mostly for medical reasons, not reproductive optionality. Embryo freezing is mostly done during IVF treatments when extra embryos are created, but also sometimes for couples who want to preserve their combined fertility, a decision which carries more considerations and legal consequences than ever.

The best time to freeze eggs, sperm, and embryos is when people are least able to afford it and usually before they've found a partner. Peak quality is in the early twenties for eggs and sperm. Social freezing, meaning freezing for nonmedical reasons, is accessible only to those with financial resources, excluding large segments of the population who would benefit. The number one concern for women in their twenties contemplating egg freezing is the cost—and rightfully so, as egg freezing patients spend between $30,000 and $40,000 in total between treatments and long-term storage. For men, it's a cheap and easy trip to a clinic or a private moment at home followed by a FedEx drop-off. There are new options, like freeze-and-share programs that allow women to freeze eggs without the upfront procedure costs if they also donate half to an egg bank. Some clinics guarantee a refund if you freeze a specific number of eggs before a certain age and cannot achieve a successful pregnancy later. New fertility insurance providers can help finance these treatments and spread the costs over years instead of charging the whole thing up front.

There are two types of freezing and thawing technologies: slow freezing and vitrification. Vitrification, which is more commonly used today, places cells into cryoprotectants, which are then plunged into liquid nitrogen, taking only seconds to freeze. The upside to vitrification is that there is no formation of ice crystals, but gametes and embryos are exposed to a high concentration of cryoprotectants. Slow freezing's gradual process is unfriendly to eggs, which are large, plump, and packed with cytoplasm and high water content. Vitrification and warming have better clinical outcomes for embryo and egg cryosurvival than slow freezing and unfreezing. They like to be frozen instantaneously and are stored in a sheet of protectants, so immediately upon thaw they can get back to the business of attracting sperm. Sperm have very little cytoplasm, which makes them more durable and easier to freeze and thaw. While all reputable clinics use vitrification for egg and embryo freezing, sperm preservation is still sometimes done via slow freezing.

EGG FREEZING

Between 2009 and 2017 there was an eighteen-times rise in the number of women who froze their eggs. Eighty-five percent of women do it not to prioritize their careers but because they cannot find a willing or desirable partner. Today's freezing and unfreezing technologies are worlds better than when they started, and only improving. But egg freezing is not a true insurance policy, or a guarantee an eventual child will be born. It is a hedge at best. There is no guarantee that eggs will survive the freezing and thawing process or will be chromosomally normal if they do. Because eggs are a single cell, testing an egg for abnormalities before it is frozen cannot be done, and knowing whether it is chromosomally normal only happens if that egg becomes an embryo. Not all embryos will make it five days to become testable either. And there is one more consideration: today, many women who freeze eggs do not ever use them.

Should I freeze my eggs?

To answer that question, here are a few more to help you consider the costs and benefits. Everyone's answers and feelings are different, so if you're contemplating these questions with friends, don't expect your reasoning to be identical. The most important bit of this exercise is complete honesty, as it is a big, expensive decision that does not always have a happy ending.

- What is my goal in freezing eggs?
- Do I want a family, and if so, how many children do I want?
- How important is it to have a biological link to my children?
- Am I at the best age to freeze eggs successfully?
- Can I afford egg freezing and the ongoing costs of preservation?

• Am I comfortable that egg freezing is not a guarantee of a future child?

There are two populations that should seriously consider egg freezing. It is usually mentioned to patients undergoing chemotherapy, radiation, or cancer-related surgery, and in those cases is sometimes covered by insurance. For trans men pursuing gender-affirming care, egg freezing doesn't always come up and is an out-of-pocket expense. The short- and long-term effects of hormone replacement therapy (HRT) on egg quality, future children, and additional impacts on fertility especially if started to suppress puberty have not been studied rigorously enough to give definitive answers.

Here is what we do know. The testosterone in HRT stops ovulation, and if the treatment stops, it's entirely possible to get pregnant even if you aren't bleeding. Babies born to parents after they stop HRT appear to be healthy, and one small study showed that the number of eggs retrieved in a transgender group was equivalent to the cisgender group, and 70 percent of the transgender group that pursued IVF afterward achieved live births. Even though the early data looks promising, it is still recommended that, if possible, egg freezing happens before starting HRT. If there is a plan to remove the ovaries or uterus, egg freezing is the only option to later maintain a genetic connection to future children. Mature eggs are produced after puberty, so trans boys and young female cancer patients can only freeze ovarian tissue before starting treatment.

Why shouldn't I freeze my eggs?

Egg freezing is not perfect. There is still a lot we do not know about freezing effects on an eventual baby nor are we likely to anytime soon. We do not know how long eggs stay viable, even in the world's most advanced, stable temperature freezer. Some women experience regret years after freezing for reasons as varied as the financial waste, having put themselves through the hormones and disruption for no reason, or not knowing what to do with frozen eggs that are not needed.

How does egg freezing work?

The egg freezing process is identical to the beginning steps of IVF:

- **Preparation:** Create a baseline of your fertility, ensure you qualify for egg freezing, find a doctor, plan financially (see if your company or insurance will contribute or line up financing if needed).
- **Stimulation:** Stimulate ovaries, monitor follicle growth, trigger egg release.
- **Retrieve:** Remove eggs under sedation, examine retrieved eggs in a lab.
- **Freeze:** Preserve mature eggs.

Once you choose a clinic and physician, the first step is performing blood tests and a pelvic ultrasound to count your antral follicles (AFC), the resting follicles that contain immature eggs that may mature and ovulate in the future. The AFC is usually done on day three of your cycle and helps to predict how many mature eggs you may get at a retrieval. Two to three weeks later you'll go over the results. The next step is more bespoke based upon the follicle count and the provider's protocols but is designed to stimulate the recruitment of a large cohort of follicles. You'll inject a series of two to three daily hormone medications at home and go in for further blood tests and ultrasounds to monitor progress. The last step before the egg retrieval is a shot that triggers eggs to reach their final stage of maturation. Thirty-six hours after the shot, the twenty-minute-long retrieval is done under general anesthesia, followed by an hour of recovery. You'll go home and rest for the remainder of the day. Some people have bloating and soreness for a few days, but the majority are back in action within a day or two. Once your eggs have been harvested, they'll be frozen immediately. If there aren't enough viable, mature eggs, you'll wait two to three months and repeat the process to build a bank of ten to twenty eggs.

What are the odds egg freezing will work for me?

One study showed that women younger than thirty-five get an aver-age of fifteen eggs per retrieval, and those older than forty-two can expect six. It usually takes multiple retrievals to build up a large-enough egg bank if you want more than one child. Here are the odds of a live birth at different ages starting with twenty frozen eggs, with a reminder that the most telling predictor of later viability is the age at which your eggs were originally frozen.

	Thirty-four years old	Thirty-seven years old	Forty-two years old
One live birth	90 percent	75 percent	37 percent
Two live births	66 percent	39 percent	7 percent
Three live births	38 percent	15 percent	1 percent

What if I move away from the clinic that is holding my eggs?

Frozen tissue can be shipped around the world, and donor eggs are often sent between clinics, in special packaging via UPS and FedEx usually. So, if you're thinking about freezing and consider-ing a move, it's possible to freeze your eggs in one clinic and have them shipped somewhere else. Same goes for embryos and sperm. Some clinics do not ship but often have a third-party service they recommend handle the logistics. Shipping internationally is usually $1,000 or more and complicated, so pick an experienced vendor who can handle the paperwork and regulations. Shipping domestically is usually under $400. As with any other shipment, things happen, so there is a very small chance that your eggs could be lost or thaw while in transit.

How do I access egg freezing if I am trans or nonbinary?

Finding gender-affirming care is critical, and it can be helpful to have someone call clinics on your behalf to ask questions related to the doctor's training and whether they have experience with people pre- and post-transition. As explained earlier, though research is still in its early days, there are specific considerations and timing for those taking or thinking about taking HRTs and for those considering surgical removal of reproductive organs.

SPERM FREEZING

Unlike women who approach egg freezing mostly for lifestyle reasons, men freeze sperm primarily if there is a medical need. Cancer patients, members of the military, and men undergoing medical procedures that could impact their sperm supply are the most frequent utilizers. Sperm freezing is offered to all transgender women before they medically transition, even under the age of eighteen, as testosterone-replacement therapy can lower sperm counts sometimes permanently.

For those reading this to learn more about frozen sperm in the context of seeking a donor, if you're thinking about joining the run on unvaccinated sperm at banks, it is wholly unnecessary and driven by the rumored and completely false negative effect the COVID-19 vaccine has on male fertility. Here it is one last time: the COVID-19 mRNA vaccine has no negative impact on male fertility. Getting COVID-19, on the other hand, does have transient negative effects on male fertility, from testicular function to sperm production and function.

How does sperm freezing work?

Unlike egg freezing, which involves precisely timed hormone injections, preserving sperm is simple: find a company that will freeze it, either online or through a local clinic, register and follow their precise instructions, get comfortable, masturbate to your material of choice, and send it in. If you are planning to freeze sperm for long-term usage, a three-month period of good lifestyle behavior should precede submitting your specimen to get the best outcome. Do not ejaculate too frequently before you submit your sample to optimize for mature sperm.

Can I freeze if my semen parameters are on the low side?

Yes, you can. Pending what's going on, you may be treated with Clomid, which is more associated with women's fertility but can also drive sperm quality back up. As you know from earlier chapters, adjusting lifestyle factors can help too. If you get this result from an at-home testing company, find a local urologist or andrologist to run in-clinic tests to see what is going on.

How long can I leave sperm frozen?

Under the right conditions, sperm can remain frozen indefinitely and later be thawed to fertilize an egg during IVF or for IUI. One study showed that there was no measurable effect on sperm frozen under five years, and only a small decrease in survival rate and impact on live birth rates when it was used in artificial insemination. Today, we're around the twenty-five-year mark on sperm thaw with no added impact on parameters. You lose around half of sperm to the freezing and unfreezing process, but since there are typically thousands if not millions in a frozen sample, unlike eggs, the loss doesn't matter that much.

How much does it cost?

That depends—some insurance covers it if there is a medical reason, and companies cover it if they offer fertility benefits, so it can cost nothing. But coverage is not broad, and for everyone else, there is an upfront cost to send and test the sample, which is a few hundred dollars, then the ongoing monthly storage cost, which varies but is around one dollar per day. The costs of cryopreservation will continue to drop as technology improves, so expect it to become more affordable in the years to come.

Is it worth it to freeze sperm?

If you're doing it for medical reasons like cancer treatments or before starting HRT, the answer is a resounding yes. If not, it depends. After looking at the nosedive happening in semen parameters coupled with age-related fertility decline, it's a good backup plan if you want to have children someday and can afford to store it. Unlike egg freezing, sperm freezing is a good insurance policy, and there are no side effects or impacts on your life leading up to giving the sample. It's also easy, so the greatest cost is financial. If you still have questions, companies and clinics employ fertility advisers who go through the pros and cons and help you decide.

EMBRYO FREEZING

Embryo freezing is another way for a single woman with a sperm donor or a couple to preserve their fertility, or if there is a medical reason to freeze. It also happens during an IVF cycle when more than one embryo is viable, since only one or two are transferred at a time. The process to freeze embryos is the same as egg freezing, with one additional step: fertilizing it with sperm before it goes into the freezer. For a long time, IVF clinics could only culture or grow cleavage-stage embryos, which were around five to eight cells and between two and three days old. Today, most embryos are frozen at the blastocyst stage, which is between five and six days after fertilization when the embryo has developed to more than seventy cells. Growing embryos longer helps to separate out the best candidates for transfer, reduces risks during genetic testing, and leads to higher birth rates. Blastocysts are one and a half times more likely to lead to a live birth than cleavage-stage embryos.

Why should I consider freezing embryos?

Frozen embryos are less delicate than eggs once fertilized, so the survival rates after freezing and unfreezing are slightly higher—95 percent for embryos versus 90 percent for eggs. You can also test frozen embryos for genetic conditions, have more information regarding their quality, and know how many true potential chances you have at pregnancy sooner than with eggs. Some people who do not have a partner decide to freeze some eggs and some embryos made with donor sperm.

Why shouldn't I freeze embryos?

There are legal and ethical questions with embryo freezing versus eggs. The first is, eggs only require one decision maker, whereas, unless you use a sperm donor, embryos require two. This dynamic can create legal problems if your current partner becomes your former. Embryos are considered property and split just like any other asset in a divorce. The question of what to do with embryos that are not needed has already figured into high-profile legal cases and inspires larger moral questions about when a human becomes a human. Parents who have fulfilled their desire for children and still have frozen embryos in storage are also faced with a choice: donation or disposal. Donation requires you to be okay with someone else raising your genetic child. For those who can't decide or can't accept the trade-offs of donating them, the storage agreement contract stipulates directions for disposal, which can be problematic too, as it is not allowed in some faiths. There are also financial considerations, as there is an additional cost to create and freeze embryos that numbers in the thousands of dollars. A growing number of providers suggest freezing eggs over embryos for fertility preservation, since the legal path is simpler in case of a breakup and outcomes are roughly equivalent. Single women almost universally choose to freeze eggs. If you're freezing extra embryos during an IVF cycle, which nearly everyone does, consider all the aforementioned information before the procedure. Most clinics will offer a fertility counselor to help navigate these questions, and some couples hire a lawyer to iron out the details of what happens should their relationship change.

What are the potential considerations for embryo freezing as it relates to reproductive rights?

During a typical IVF or freezing cycle, multiple embryos are made and frozen since not all will be viable for transfer. The possibility of personhood statutes, which seek to legally establish that an embryo has constitutional rights, is a serious legal consideration. Individual states have tried and failed to pass personhood legislation since most voters recognize that the ruling negatively impacts infertility care and birth control too. If these laws pass in your state, ask your clinic for their guidance, and if you should move your embryos or seek care in a nearby state where this is not the case.

TISSUE PRESERVATION

Until 2019, ovarian tissue preservation (OTP) was considered experimental. Now it is indicated for cancer patients (although not for leukemia patients, as the risk of reseeding the cancer is too high) or trans men undergoing gender-affirming surgery. OTP is usually combined with egg freezing and is what it sounds like: egg-producing tissue from the ovary is removed under anesthesia, through a laparoscopic procedure, then frozen. The procedure requires a few days of recovery time. When it's time for the tissue to be reimplanted, the tissue is thawed and placed near the remaining ovarian tissue. Live birth rates after tissue reintroduction are around 30 percent, and one-third of those required IVF. The downside is that OTP requires two separate surgeries, but unlike egg freezing it does not require hormone injections or any other protocols leading up to it. For cancer patients, there is a risk that the ovary contains cancer cells. And not all the immature eggs that are removed with the ovary will survive. The effects of a single piece of implanted tissue can last between four and eight years, and when a second surgery with another piece of preserved tissue is performed, the clock starts over.

For men, testicular tissue preservation is done for those undergoing treatments that will render them infertile, for those who cannot freeze sperm, or for those undergoing IVF. It carries the same risk of containing cancer cells and the practice is still experimental; to date there have been no live births from frozen testicular tissue.

There is one other exciting area of fertility preservation. Ovarian tissue preservation with later reintroduction premenopause may add years to women's reproductive life spans. Reproductive longevity research seeks to halt ovarian aging, giving women the ability to start a family whenever they like and help those faced with premature menopause. Ovaries age up to five times faster than any other organ in the body, which is often the cause of infertility and a longer span of poor health later in life. Even though human life spans have doubled in the past two centuries, the age at which women go through menopause has not changed with it. Beyond having babies later, which is not really the point, reproductive longevity therapies could reduce the negative effects on cardiovascular, cognitive, and immune health that happen because of menopause too.

Fertility Preservation Wrap-Up

Sperm freezing	**What to know:** A great, relatively inexpensive option for any man under thirty-five who is worried about his fertility. Should be considered before cancer and HRT treatments and gender-affirming surgeries if there is a wish for a genetic child in the future. **Cost:** Total cost for semen analysis, freezing, and one year of storage is under $1,000.
Egg freezing	**What to know:** It does not guarantee a baby, and most women don't use them later. The best time to freeze eggs is when you are under thirty-five. **Cost:** Between drugs, retrievals, and storage it's between $30,000 and $40,000 on average. Fertility financing is an option to pay over time.
Embryo freezing	**What to know:** Embryos (no matter how or when they are created) are considered an asset in a breakup, so consider speaking to a lawyer before IVF or embryo freezing. **Cost:** Most of the time they are done as part of an IVF cycle, so there are several thousand dollars of fees related to storage and culturing the embryos. If it's done outside of IVF, costs are slightly higher than egg freezing.
Ovarian tissue preservation	**What to know:** This experimental procedure is usually done for prepubescent female cancer patients or trans boys who are not old enough to freeze eggs. Testicular freezing is even earlier in development. **Cost:** Insurance in some cases cover it. If it's out of pocket, surgery starts around $10,000 and yearly storage costs are $300 to $500.

Chapter 14

FERTILITY TREATMENT AND ASSISTED REPRODUCTION

Dealing with infertility and today's options to start a family

In 1455, "Henry the Impotent," the King of Castile, married Princess Joana of Portugal. Six years later, their daughter was born amid court whispers that she could not possibly be his biological child. The reason for his rumored impotence was lost to history, though it's hypothesized that he had erectile dysfunction due to a tumor. While we will never know for sure how she was conceived, it was the first time an attempt at artificial insemination is mentioned in history books. Three hundred years later, the first assisted reproduction procedure was performed in London by John Hunter, the founder of scientific surgery. He directed a patient with a congenital defect in his penis to collect semen in a warmed syringe post-sex so it could be injected into his wife's vagina. Nine months later, they welcomed a child. Gregory Pincus, famed for developing the birth control pill, was the first to successfully achieve in vitro fertilization in any species, in this case, rabbits. Unfortunately, Pincus's breakthrough happened in 1934, around the time that Aldous Huxley's *Brave New World*, which featured test tube babies, hit bookshelves. International backlash ensued, culminating in Dr. Pincus's dismissal from Harvard and a brief stint as a janitor to make ends meet. Yet he persisted and his work informed Patrick Steptoe, Robert Edwards, and Jean Purdy, the scientific trio behind Louise Brown, the first human IVF baby. Since her groundbreaking birth in 1978, an estimated eight million IVF babies have been born, and more than two and a half million IVF cycles are performed each year.

Technological advances in fertility treatment are transforming the industry, and the culture of secrecy around it is falling away too. Global news reports circulated of a seventy-four-year-old Indian woman who delivered twin girls via IVF after trying to start a family for fifty-seven years. Neil Patrick Harris and David Burtka are each biologically related to one of their fraternal twins, who were carried by a surrogate. First Lady Michelle Obama conceived her daughters via IVF. And after health complications, Kim Kardashian used a gestational carrier for her last two children.

The goal with fertility treatment is to start with less invasive, inexpensive treatments before moving on—there is no "just do IVF." Pending the diagnosis, your doctor may try medications or change lifestyle factors before jumping into any assisted reproduction treatments (ART) like IUI or IVF. Third-party reproduction is a variation of ART that can involve using donor gametes, a surrogate (has a genetic relationship to the baby and carries it), or gestational carrier (has no genetic relationship and carries the baby), or a combination. The exact course of treatment depends on how long you've tried to conceive, your and your partner's ages, health, genetic, and fertility profiles—and what you can afford.

Cost and access are the biggest barriers to fertility treatment the world over, with few exceptions. In the United States, private insurance and Medicaid rarely, if ever, cover it. Some states have laws requiring insurers to pay for IVF, so check your geography. Denmark, home to the world's biggest sperm bank, also counts itself as a destination for fertility tourists. IVF is responsible for 10 percent of all live births there, and three fresh IVF transfers or five cycles are publicly funded for patients between eighteen and forty years old. The United Kingdom's National Health Service (NHS)–funded IVF is offered to women under forty-three but there are conditions. They must try to conceive for two years or have twelve cycles of IUI to qualify. Even if a woman meets that criterion, a local clinical commissioning group has the final say. Ultimately, the population with the most coverage (outside of the Danes) are those with private insurance and fertility benefits. They are, paradoxically, the ones that need financial assistance the least.

Calculating exactly how much it will cost to pursue fertility treatments is difficult. The expense varies based on the medications or procedures a provider suggests in advance of ART, then the number of treatments or cycles needed to produce a successful pregnancy as well as any drugs or IVF add-ons, which differ clinic to clinic.

Here is an example of how this plays out. Women aged thirty-five and younger generally respond well to IVF drugs and have a simpler, less expensive template protocol. One is known as minimal stimulation IVF (mini IVF or min stim), and it uses an oral medication (Clomid) versus injections before an egg retrieval. The reason min stim doesn't work as well for women older than thirty-five is that as age increases, so does the amount of drugs needed to stimulate the ovaries to produce follicles. Older ovaries are less responsive and less likely to produce quality eggs that survive to a live birth.

There are variations in the ways clinicians administer drugs too; each has a preferred method. Regimens can be performed in the clinic or at home with a nurse at an additional expense but most commonly are self-administered or done by a partner. Pending all these options and the bevy of add-ons clinics offer, there is a cost to every additional drug, step, protocol, and person involved in your treatment.

Highly educated Caucasian and Asian professionals have the most access to fertility care because they are more likely to work at companies that provide fertility benefits. As education level and income drop so does participation in fertility treatments. LGBTQ+ individuals do not meet the official definition of infertility, and although this is changing, the result is they do not always qualify for services, including fertility preservation. It also can be difficult to find gender-affirming care or to identify a surrogate, which is still not legal for gay couples in some parts of the world.

There is another open secret in the ART industry that colors where people seek treatment—and if they are treated at all. Some providers turn away patients whose outcomes are unlikely to be successful. The reasons range from age, BMI, to underlying health conditions, and, in most cases, there is nothing you can do to change their minds. Accepting a poor-prognosis patient and their money isn't exactly ethical, even with informed consent (though that is still a subject of debate). But denying care if there is little chance of success (even if the patient accepts that risk) benefits the clinic too, as treatment outcomes are publicly reported to SART and the CDC. If one clinic refuses treatment, ensure you understand why, and try another if you are willing to assume the financial and emotional risks. Know that if you do, it may involve a compromise, like using donor gametes for IVF, and that some clinics that take on high-risk patients will have lower outcome data that reflects it.

Before we jump into the options, there are predictable emotional triggers if things are not happening on the pregnancy timeline you'd like. The holidays are difficult, as many prospective parents use gatherings to share good news with family and friends. Reaching the end of March without success means that you won't welcome a baby in that calendar year. Finding yourself surrounded by friends who (seemingly) sneezed and got pregnant can feel unfair too. You may not feel up to going to baby showers, and that's okay. Fertility treatments and pregnancy are personal, and if you want to keep the circle of those in the know small, do it. If sharing is your jam, great. Just be prepared to share bad news if it happens. If you're on this journey with a partner, talk about how you're feeling, openly and often. And not to plug it again, but therapy should be a standard of care for anyone navigating infertility or undergoing fertility treatment. No matter how great your family and friends and partner are, there will, at some point, be things you cannot or do not want to say out loud to them.

LOW-INTERVENTION FERTILITY TREATMENTS

Medications

If you aren't ovulating, or if the issue is unknown, your provider may suggest fertility medications. Clomiphene citrate (Clomid) is the most routine prescription for ovulatory issues, as it blocks estrogen and tells your brain to release more of the hormones that trigger egg production. If Clomid doesn't work, there are hormone injections— FSH, HCG, and human menopausal gonadotropin (HMG), among them—that can have the same effect. Suppressing ovulation is sometimes necessary with conditions like endometriosis, so drugs including oral contraceptives or gNRH agonists will be prescribed in that case.

For men, Clomid is sometimes prescribed to stimulate the production of testosterone and sperm, especially for those with low testosterone levels or nonobstructive azoospermia. Another common male fertility drug is anastrozole, which reduces estrogen levels and raises testosterone to treat low libido and erectile dysfunction and increase sperm count. HCG injections are used if nothing else is working, and treatment involves two to three visits per week to a physician for injections. But it can help with sperm production and raises the likelihood of a successful sperm retrieval in men with nonobstructive azoospermia.

Timed intercourse

Think of timed intercourse as pinpointing your exact fertile window with tools beyond ovulation-prediction kits or cycle tracking.

Typically, you'll start with hormone testing, then visit your provider for ultrasound monitoring of follicular development. When the time is right, you'll have sex every day or every other day during that precisely timed window. Sometimes monitoring is all it takes, or it can be coupled with medications like Clomid or hormone injections if you need help with ovulation. If the goal is to monitor a cycle and produce more mature eggs, timed intercourse with the same fertility drugs used during IUI or IVF stimulation cycles can address it. While some ob-gyns can manage this process, it may be time to pursue more specialized treatment with a RE as approaches and training count.

Intracervical insemination (ICI)

Sometimes referred to as the turkey-baster method, its technical name is intracervical insemination (ICI). ICI is designed to deposit sperm into the vagina near the cervix via a plastic syringe, or a cervical cap or menstrual disc is used to keep the semen close to the cervix and mucus, preventing backflow into the vagina. It can work for lesbian couples, single women, and gay men working with a surrogate, and is increasingly popular with heterosexual couples who cannot cope with another month of timed sex. Please do not use kitchen utensils—there are companies that offer at-home insemination kits that are FDA-cleared and make it easy and more likely to work. Targeting the fertile window, gather a fresh sperm sample, through masturbation or a collection condom, or a frozen specimen from a sperm bank. Whether freshly ejaculated or thawed (follow the bank's instructions), either transfer semen into the cervical cap and insert into your vagina, or fill the syringe with semen, lie on your back, insert the syringe into your vagina like a tampon until it stops, and ready, aim, fire at your cervix. Staying horizontal right after ICI is recommended, so gravity doesn't interfere with the sperm finding their way to an egg. While IUI and ICI have somewhat similar approaches, ICI simulates what happens during sex and the insertion stops at the cervix, not all the way into the uterus. IUI costs around four times as ICI, but efficacy is only marginally better, even though sperm used for IUI is "washed," leaving only healthy sperm to be injected into the uterus. This makes ICI a worthy consideration for any couple dealing with unexplained infertility before progressing to more expensive treatments.

ASSISTED REPRODUCTION TREATMENTS

Intrauterine insemination (IUI)

IUI is used in the case of low sperm counts or abnormal sperm parameters, hostile cervical mucus, vaginismus (a condition that causes involuntary vaginal constrictions), and unexplained infertility. It is also used by single women or gay men working with a surrogate. If IVF is financially out of reach and the issue is male factor infertility, IUI with donor sperm is an option too.

Known as donor insemination, artificial insemination, or alternative insemination, IUI works by injecting sperm directly into the uterus around the time of ovulation. Think of it as a cheat code, positioning sperm at the perfect time and place to fertilize an egg as it descends. Like ICI, IUI is a low-tech procedure, but instead of doing it at home, it is done in-office using a speculum. The prep for IUI starts with tracking your fertile window and monitoring appointments as needed. IUI can also involve oral medications like Clomid or hormone injections. The closer IUI is done to ovulation the better. A sperm sample must go through a washing process to remove nonliving and poorly functioning sperm, white blood cells, and seminal fluid components like prostaglandins, which can cause painful uterine contractions. After the semen sample is prepared, it is placed into a large catheter (à la bucatini pasta) and inserted into the uterus. At-home IUI is a terrible idea for many reasons, the main two being that putting unwashed semen into the uterus causes uterine contractions and accessing internal body cavities so intimately is best left to professionals with sterile instruments in sterile environments.

A common IUI question is outside of cost, is there a compelling, evidence-based reason to start with IUI versus going straight to IVF? When the problem is male-factor infertility it is a great place to begin as IUI can increase the number of sperm that make it into the fallopian tube by one thousand. It is less invasive and time intensive and requires no drugs or extended time frames to start unless medications are needed to help mature or ovulate eggs. It does not require anesthesia or surgery, just a sperm sample, a known fertile window, and several office visits. The success rate is between 5 and 20 percent per cycle, and the highest likelihood of success is during the first three to four treatments. If you were excited by the prospect of freezing multiple embryos with IVF, IUI does not provide that option.

In Vitro Fertilization (IVF)

Between 1 and 3 percent of all births in the United States and Europe happen via IVF. The rates are close to 7 percent in Japan, and higher in other areas of the world. For all its evolution, IVF is still a very bespoke process. Testing protocols, culturing techniques, and opinions vary based on geography and by clinic and clinician. But things may be changing. Companies are removing the human element with smart petri dishes that allow less handling during embryo culturing. AI can ingest data from millions of IVF cycles to create more personalized treatment options, like precisely pinpointing the timing of the trigger shot during ovarian stimulation. Many top clinics feature physiologic IVF lab circuits, which simulate the environment and oxygen levels in the uterus while embryos are handled. Others allow patients to monitor their developing embryos via apps. And thanks to more open reporting and conversation within the industry, shared best practices should lead to better, more consistent treatment methodologies and outcomes.

IVF is performed in couples experiencing infertility—after failed IUI, and in the case of health conditions like ovulatory disorders, blocked fallopian tubes, recurrent miscarriage, and male-factor infertility like low sperm count. It is rare to go straight to IVF without trying low intervention

treatments first, except for addressing the risk of passing on genetic disorders or for single parents or couples using a gestational carrier. IVF is
invasive, and the ten to twelve days of hormone shots required to stimulate egg production before retrieval cause side effects like irritation, bloating, and moodiness. And the anxiety related to the big question—will it
work?—makes IVF an emotionally draining process for everyone.

A single IVF cycle describes an egg retrieval and an embryo transfer.
Pending the outcome of the first cycle, the retrieval or transfer is sometimes repeated. All IVF cycles start with stimulating the ovaries to grow
eggs. Minimum stimulation relies on oral medications, and a full stimulation process is done via a series of hormone injections, primarily of
gonadotropins that contain FSH and LH. Birth control pills are almost
always prescribed before a retrieval to help the ovaries better respond
to the stimulation medications and allow the cycle to be scheduled for
a convenient time. 36 hours before the egg retrieval, an injection of
HCG known as the trigger shot is given to stimulate the final stages of
egg maturation. While you are anesthetized, eggs are retrieved via a thin
needle guided by ultrasound, then isolated in the embryology lab where
they are mixed with sperm. When they fertilize successfully, the resulting embryos are grown in a lab and, once matured, given a grade to
designate its potential based upon characteristics like fragmentation and
total number of cells. Then it is transferred into the uterus or frozen.

In a fresh transfer, embryos are placed inside the uterus between
three and five days after the retrieval in the hope that they will implant, so estrogen levels will still be high, which can change the quality
of the endometrium. A frozen embryo transfer can happen any time,
even years later, and involves the additional steps of freezing and thawing embryos. Only frozen embryos can be genetically tested, which
is one reason most IVF cycles now use them. Embryos with normal
chromosome numbers or no known genetic defects are selected and
transferred later. Another benefit is that the endometrium has time to
recover from the hormone stimulation before transfer, and the timeline more closely mimics a natural menstrual cycle. For women with

PCOS, using frozen embryos lowers the risk of ovarian overstimulation syndrome, and live birth rates are higher. But there are still unanswered questions. Vitrification is a huge advance in cryopreservation, but the potential for embryo injury via cryoprotectant agents is not zero. Fresh transfers are also sometimes done as backup if embryos aren't developing well enough to go through the freezing process. Another possibility is a mixed cycle where one or two fresh embryos are implanted, and the rest are frozen for a later attempt.

Another nuance to transfer is development time. The cleavage stage of development happens two to three days after fertilization, and blastocyst is five or six days. Because blastocysts have had more time to develop, they consist of far more cells and are differentiated into two distinct parts: the inner cell mass, which becomes the fetus, and the trophectoderm, which becomes extra embryonic tissue and the placenta. Cleavage stage embryos are just eight to sixteen totipotent cells, meaning they are not yet differentiated; blastocysts are differentiated and typically between seventy to one hundred cells. Embryo transfer is mostly done at the blastocyst phase, as cell culture media has advanced such that embryos can be grown safely for longer. Outcomes appear to be better waiting before implantation, and anyone who wants genetic testing must wait until the blastocyst stage anyway, so there is less risk to the embryo. If you are unable to grow embryos to a blastocyst stage, a fresh transfer may be done with a three-day cleavage-stage embryo.

Historically, multiples (twins, triplets, etc.) were more common to parents who used ART (though multiple embryo transfers are increasingly rare) and there was a higher risk of preterm birth because it is associated with multiples. Today's ART best practices preference singleton births, but even among singletons, the rate of preterm birth is almost double in ART babies, perhaps because parents are typically older or have existing health conditions that drive them to fertility treatments. The odds of a single IVF cycle working also vary based on age. Typical success rates are 20 to 35 percent per embryo transfer to achieve a live birth. But there is more nuance depending on the cause of infertility and how many healthy embryos are created after each retrieval. Couples with embryo-quality issues, for example, may require multiple egg retrievals to make a single healthy embryo that implants the first time. Other couples may be able to generate healthy embryos from a single retrieval but need multiple transfers to get one to stick. If it doesn't work the first time, the drug protocol is usually tweaked before another attempt.

Intracytoplasmic sperm injection (ICSI)

The advent of this procedure has taken the world of male fertility by storm. ICSI is a technique developed for men whose sperm parameters don't meet the needs of IVF. Unlike traditional fertilization during IVF, which requires thousands of sperm, ICSI requires just one sperm for each egg. It has huge advantages, namely incredible precision in choosing the most viable single sperm. The ability to select a normally shaped and swimming sperm is why it is now used in three out of every four IVF procedures even when the underlying reason for pursuing assisted reproduction is not male factor infertility. While some patients benefit—especially those undergoing preimplantation genetic testing or those who are using frozen eggs—ICSI maximizes but does not guarantee fertilization, nor does it universally raise the live birth rate, the metric in IVF that truly matters.

ICSI is not a therapy, and its availability and efficacy has led clinicians to care less about the specifics of a semen analysis; merely the presence or absence of enough viable sperm is enough information. That puts the weight of managing fertility back onto women, since there is no similar treatment for eggs. Within the research world, ICSI diminished the amount of attention and research investigation sperm get, which could help avoid these issues altogether. If you're undergoing IVF with no male-factor infertility or genetic testing of embryos in play and ICSI is advised, ask why. Data for use of ICSI indicates that fertilization rates for non-male factor are equal (perhaps slightly better) to when it is not used, but ICSI is not free, and is unnecessarily applied to treatments in a conspicuous number of cases.

Preimplantation genetic testing

Before the 1990s, the only way to mitigate genetic risks in embryos was limited to chorionic villus sampling (CVS) and amniocentesis well into a pregnancy. Now, it's common to test IVF embryos during the blastocyst stage before they are implanted. There are two types of genetic testing: preimplantation genetic screening for abnormal chromosome number (PGT-A) and preimplantation genetic testing for individual diseases (PGT-M). It takes between one and two weeks to get results, so after the cell sample is taken, the embryo is frozen until results come back. If you are going through a fresh transfer, there are other ways to assess and select embryos, like cleavage rates and examining morphological characteristics under the microscope.

PGT-A looks for embryonic aneuploidy, or an irregular number of chromosomes, which can cause miscarriage, implantation failure, and less successful overall IVF outcomes. Caused by DNA damage, errors during cell division, and fertilization errors, it increases the likelihood of chromosomal instability within an embryo. For women older than thirty-five, there's roughly a 50 percent incidence of aneuploidy in embryos produced during IVF, and that number increases with age. As the fertilized egg divides and multiplies into cells, errors that occur down the line can be replicated. But the normal cells might have a competitive advantage over the abnormal cells, leading most of the cells in the embryo to have the correct number of chromosomes. Other times, there may be abnormal or normal cells present even if the sample indicates otherwise, since so few are removed for testing.

We're also learning that some abnormal cells may self-correct over time, which means that clinics may be disposing of embryos that may otherwise develop normally. These are known as mosaic embryos, which contain differing percentages of normal and abnormal cells that develop after fertilization. Mosaic embryos sometimes grow normally and result in full-term, healthy births. Until recently, transferring a mosaic embryo was only done in special circumstances, but there is a push in the industry for further research. As a result of this uncertainty, PGT-A testing is still under scrutiny, and some scientists question if it's a good idea to do it at all.

PGT-M is used to detect more than four hundred single-gene disorders and is done if one or both biological parents are carriers for a condition. Most single-gene disorders require both parents to be carriers, and in those cases the odds are 25 percent that the condition will be passed down. But for conditions that require only one defective gene, the odds of it being present in an embryo go up to 50 percent, so it's important to test.

Genetic testing is low-risk, but it isn't zero, so the question of whether to do it lies primarily in the hands of your RE and genetic counselor. They will help you interpret results and the resulting risk profile if any issues are uncovered. Genetic testing isn't universally recommended yet, as there is still a bias toward favorable prognosis, it's not free, there is a risk of false-positive results, and the possibility of embryo damage. However, when an IVF cycle fails and testing was not performed, it is usually the first thing blamed.

IVF ADD-ONS

Some clinics allow you to treat your embryos to classical music as they develop in their petri dish, or watch their development through an app—for an extra fee. IVF add-ons vary in purpose, and the evidence in many cases is lacking. Though some experts argue that, just like supplements, regulation of these procedures would delay potentially life-changing results for patients, most call for real evidence before they should ever be presented. The FDA only requires formal regulatory review when "human cellular and tissue-based products are manipulated to a more-than-minimal degree," and so far, none of these add-ons meet that criteria. No criteria means no formal review. Until more research is conducted, if you are presented with any of these protocols, ask how they bring real value to an already expensive treatment before you commit.

Endometrial scratching

To show how little the fertility industry agrees on best practices, meet endometrial scratching (ES). Offered more frequently in Australia, New Zealand, and the United Kingdom than the United States, ES is a practice that can be done before implantation during IVF. It's an intentional injury done to the endometrium performed as an endometrial biopsy or curettage prior to embryo transfer to enhance its receptivity. It came into fashion more than two decades ago when Israeli doctors noticed that women who had undergone a uterine-lining biopsy appeared to have higher pregnancy rates. While ES rates are falling, thanks to the lack of evidence that supports its use, it is still sometimes offered if there is implantation failure. It's also reported more commonly as a last line of defense after several failed IVF rounds, mostly for psychological reasons. And that benefit is accurate: half the participants polled in one study said it reduced distress and a third claimed it offered hope. But as with everything it must be weighed with the pain, discomfort, cost, and inconvenience of the procedure.

HCG injections

If you've ever taken a pregnancy test, HCG is the hormone that causes that second pink line. Its normal function is to support egg development in the ovaries and stimulate the release of eggs during ovulation, making this novel approach to improving IVF outcomes somewhat intuitive on its face. Done by injecting a synthetic form of HCG (IC-HCG) through a catheter around the time of embryo transfer, the procedure is thought to stimulate and improve the endometrium. So, is it worth it? The evidence is mixed. If you are undergoing a cleavage-stage transfer it appears to improve the live birth rate. For those undergoing blastocyst transfer, there simply isn't enough evidence, and there is nothing to support a reduction in miscarriage rates irrespective of embryo stage at transfer.

Interestingly, the biggest benefit might be to women with endometriosis, as it improves pregnancy rates in those undergoing frozen embryo transfer.

Immune suppression

When a human embryo enters a woman's body, it contains foreign genes from a father, and for many years scientists believed that was why a woman's body seemed to be in an immune-suppressed state during pregnancy. Reality is more nuanced than that, but this belief is why in this add-on treatment, steroids, IV immunoglobulin, and powerful antibodies are administered to suppress a patient's immune system. This all falls into the category of reproductive immunology, which some providers support and others do not. The hope is that it will be in a weakened-enough state that it will not attack the embryo. And there is no evidence that it works or increases the chances of a live birth except in the case of patients with autoimmune disorders. There is, however, evidence of harm as these drugs can cause side effects like fever, infection, mood changes, weight gain, headaches, and even diabetes and kidney failure, and for the fetus premature birth and growth restriction. When corticosteroid use continues during the first trimester, it is linked to congenital abnormalities like cleft lip and palate in infants.

Embryo glue

Though it isn't technically glue, the process of embryo gluing is thought to make the embryo more adherent to the walls of the uterus. The "glue" is mostly hyaluronic acid (which you may know from your face serum but is a sugar that occurs naturally in the body). It is added to the embryo-transfer medium and the embryo is dipped into it right before implantation. So, does it work? Research is weak but concludes that it may very slightly improve the number of live births, clinical pregnancies, and multiple pregnancies. It does not help miscarriage rates or other adverse events.

Polygenic risk scores

No matter which side you're on regarding polygenic risk scores (PRS)—huge potential, bad science, or thinly veiled eugenics—if you talk to anyone in this field, you'll be met with strongly worded reasons that you are wrong. PRS or genetic risk scores provide the relative risk that you will inherit or pass on a disease. The results are a risk mitigation measure—not a certainty. PRS is a powerful tool, but it cannot give an exact likelihood that a disease will manifest, nor can it give a timeline of its progression.

While it is sometimes marketed to couples before they conceive to determine whether based on their risk factors, pursuing assisted reproduction beats natural conception, the primary use case for PRS today is for embryo selection during an IVF cycle.

Why, you may be asking, is PRS one of the most rage-inducing topics in reproductive medicine? Because it assesses polygenic conditions like type 2 diabetes or heart disease, which do not occur on a single gene—they can pop up in hundreds if not thousands. Scientists must look at the DNA sequences of a large population with the disease and compare it to a population without it to find the most common differences. The data is then converted into a risk score that tells prospective parents how genetically similar the embryo is to others with the condition. Proponents claim PRS increases the probability the embryo selected will be viable and high quality. Naysayers have issues both moral and technical, and claim, because of the lack of absolute certainty PRS analyses provide, the technique shouldn't be used for embryo selection.

There is a lot we don't understand about the impacts of meddling with genetic variation and PRS cannot account for all unknowns or epigenetic changes. PRS does not factor in the environment that a child will be born into, or lifestyle choices that could activate (or not) that disease. There also is no way to know if a treatment or cure for the diseases prospective parents wish to avoid will exist by the time their child grows up. Maybe it won't even matter! Most genetic data sets consist primarily of adults of European ancestry, so PRS may not be accurate across all ethnic groups either. We don't know if genetic data from adults translates directly to embryos since so much development hinges on environment. PRS doubters also cite pleiotropy, or the phenomena in which a single gene affects multiple traits, as another unknown. Selecting for one positive trait could have unintended consequences, like accidentally increasing the risk of another negative trait. And the stickiest ethical issue of all: the belief that the ability to select embryos by traits will lead parents to opt for those with the highest intelligence, attractiveness, and height.

PRS isn't going away. One company leaped over the challenges of accurately sequencing an embryo's entire genome (since an embryo by its very nature is just a few cells) by reconstructing the missing bits from full sequences of both parents' DNA. For a blastocyst, the reconstructed genome match was 98 percent. So, although the technology isn't perfect, it is something you may be offered if you pursue IVF and want to mitigate possible genetic risks. If you're thinking about PRS, consider starting with carrier screening and genetic testing for inherited Mendelian disorders first.

USING DONOR GAMETES AND THIRD-PARTY REPRODUCTION

When IVF treatments fail because eggs or sperm are not viable, the next step is to use donor gametes. In other cases, if there are physiological reasons a woman cannot carry a pregnancy to term, or for LGBTQ+ or single prospective parents, a gestational carrier or surrogate is used. While all three routes provide a path for more people to become parents, using donor gametes and carriers can be complicated. There is no universal egg and sperm bank, nor is it possible to do a Google search of every available bank. Each bank requires its own search based upon the specific criteria parents want, from IQ to race to number of languages spoken and height. And because so many of these criteria are the same, there is a shortage of sperm and eggs that meet it.

Donors and carriers are categorized as known (someone you know in the real world or a donor at a bank who disclosed their identity) or unknown, meaning the donor wished to remain anonymous, though that is increasingly uncommon. For known donors, conversations should explore how and when to tell the child and any family or community as well as setting boundaries for the donor's involvement in the child's life.

When using anonymous donor gametes, a consideration is how or when to tell a future child they are not biologically related. In the past, doctors discouraged telling children about their genetic origins. Now the guidance has flipped so they are not surprised later in life and their conception story becomes part of their identity from the start. Conversations may also include navigating the lack of family history or medical information in the future should there be an emergency. Some of the same privacy and boundary questions apply to a carrier relationship, especially if it is a family member or friend. Carriers who you hire from agencies are structured relationships that require more paperwork and legal agreements. (And money!)

There is another consideration for prospective LGBTQ+ parents. Parent is a legal status. The legal definition depends on where you live, as every state has different laws around how they recognize it. A marriage, civil union, or domestic partnership is not enough to earn parent status under the marriage presumption, which assumes that a child is biologically related to both people in that relationship. In most states, the parent who did not carry the baby, or non-gestational carrier, must adopt them after birth. Reciprocal IVF, when one woman supplies the egg and the other carries the pregnancy, is an option for lesbian couples, and gives both an opportunity to feel more intimately involved. But even there, the parent who did not carry the pregnancy must adopt the baby, even though they are genetically related. So, if you are considering IUI or IVF, speak to a lawyer who specializes in these issues before you get started.

Using donor eggs

It is normal that, eventually, the ovaries are done producing eggs that can result in a healthy pregnancy, usually between ages forty and forty-five. Egg donation is necessary in this case, and for women born without ovaries, or whose ovaries have been removed. For other women, endometriosis, cancer treatment, an inherited genetic condition, or another unknown reason can trigger a halt sooner. Egg donation is also used to avoid passing down inherited conditions, or if eggs are found not to be viable for other reasons while undergoing IVF treatments. In these cases, donor eggs give women the option to experience pregnancy, give birth, and grow a family.

Some women choose to become egg donors because they have a friend or family member who struggled with fertility, or they wanted to learn more about their genetic backgrounds thanks to the rigorous screenings they must undergo to qualify. Others do it for financial reasons, as compensation starts between $10,000 to $15,000 per donation cycle. Women undergoing IVF treatments can agree to donate extra eggs to infertile patients, though the practice is perceived as coercive, especially if a discount on IVF treatment is offered. Freeze-and-share arrangements provide the procedure for free if a woman donates half of her eggs. Universally, donors don't pay for anything, and the list of qualifying tests and screenings is long. The minimum requirement is that they must be a healthy woman between the ages of twenty-one and thirty-four with a BMI less than thirty who does not smoke or use recreational drugs. Once a donor meets that qualification, they must go through extensive medical tests and psychological screenings, and sign legal documents related to the donation. Though the risks from donating eggs are low, donors often get a supplemental insurance policy to cover medical care required after an egg retrieval (e.g., ovarian hyperstimulation syndrome).

Intended parents have a choice: fresh or frozen eggs. Frozen eggs sourced from egg banks are more common; fresh eggs are rarely shipped unless they are going to someone in the same city. This decision will be left to your fertility specialist and your timing, though it's worth considering how many children you'd eventually like to have. If it's just one or two, a frozen egg bank can work. If you'd like to preserve a genetic relationship between future children and plan to have three or more, the cost per egg is close to the same as the full cycle with a fresh donor. Six is usually the number of mature eggs purchased at a time. Frozen eggs are available for use immediately, meaning as soon as they are shipped from the bank to your clinic they can be fertilized and transferred. But the supply of frozen eggs is more limited than fresh, which means your choice of donor is too. Fresh eggs require a prepayment to secure the donor, then when the donor undergoes a retrieval, all the resulting eggs from that cycle will be shipped immediately to your clinic for fertilization and transfer. The time from selection to retrieval is usually between sixty and ninety days. Either method is expensive: the cost to use a donor egg is an average of $15,000 and can exceed $25,000 for premium donors. Some clinics allow intended parents to split the costs and resulting eggs from a retrieval with other families.

What makes a premium donor? Ethnicity and family heritage are two criteria that can be particularly difficult for intended parents to match and they drive up costs. Women of Asian descent, particularly those who are 100 percent full ethnicity of Chinese, Korean, or Japanese heritage are in high demand. Fertility issues are not discussed openly in Asian culture, and there is a strong connection to family history and genetics, which can mean that many people are not open to being an egg or sperm donor. Middle Eastern and East Indian egg donors are hard to find, as certain religious practices common in these regions do not support these procedures and explaining them to more traditionally minded family members can be difficult. High IQ and an Ivy League education are also popular, as are donors who share physical and personality traits and interests like music or athletic pursuits with intended parents.

While most cultures have a laissez-faire attitude toward sperm donation, egg donation carries more weight. Perhaps due to eggs' relative scarcity compared to sperm. Or because women are born with all they will ever have. Certainly, because the process to retrieve and use eggs is an invasive and time-consuming surgical procedure versus walking into a room with a cup. But there is also blatant sexism around the perceived emotional relationship women have with eggs versus men and their sperm, which led to the belief that a financial incentive is somehow less ethical. For that reason, altruism weighs heavily during the psych screening.

Using donor sperm

Although the first recorded instance of donor insemination happened in the United States in the 1880s, the real breakthrough was in 1949, when glycerol was used to protect sperm during freezing and unfreezing. Between 2015 and 2017, an estimated 440,986 women in the United States used donor sperm to conceive. It's only an estimate because the procedure has always been secretive. The profile of those who use donor sperm are primarily white, city-dwelling, college-educated, older, high-income women, and more specifically, 60 percent are gay women, 20 percent are single mothers by choice, and 20 percent are heterosexual couples. When heterosexual couples use donor sperm, it's usually because there is a complete absence of sperm or very low sperm count, a heritable disease, or if the vas deferens are blocked after a vasectomy or due to a congenital malformation. The reason donor sperm is not used as frequently by heterosexual couples is because ICSI only requires one viable sperm, and sperm can be extracted directly from the testicles using a surgical procedure if needed.

What do people want in a sperm donor? Key search terms are *young* and *highly educated*. Physically attractive donor profiles are sometimes posted on a bank's website in the morning and completely gone by lunchtime. The donor supply was dire before the pandemic, and with the increase in demand that period of isolation drove, an unregulated cottage industry of donors popped up in private social media groups. On the internet, donors do not need to live by the same FDA-regulated rules. Traditional sperm banks limit donors to between twenty-five and thirty families. Not so on the Wild West intertubes where men often do not follow these limits. However, they offer prospective families something sperm banks can't: their identities. Even though it's possible to identify an anonymous donor or biological siblings using consumer genetic companies, sperm banks do not allow families to know their donor's real identity at purchase. While this sounds appealing, knowing poses legal risks related to custody and child support. There are other risks to getting sperm from an unknown source, namely that they don't always disclose medical and genetic conditions that can lead to health problems that parents did not expect.

FINDING A FERTILITY CLINIC

Fertility treatment is one part detective work, one part treatment. The clinic you use impacts the outcome, and finding one is a maze of references, internet searches, and budgeting decisions. The easiest way to choose a provider is through your existing medical provider, or a referral that has firsthand experience with the clinic, like a friend or colleague. The other is to look for reviews and information online. Key topics to dig into beyond clinical outcomes are patient experience, communication, and responsiveness. State-by-state and clinic-specific data is available on the CDC website at www.cdc.gov/art or www.SART.org. One important distinction: SART includes cycle-start information while the CDC only reports outcome statistics for completed cycles, so the data sets on SART are more extensive.

When evaluating outcome data, know that a clinic's success rates may vary year over year based on the number of cycles they perform. Those that do more cycles have more consistent stats over time. An individual clinic's success is tied to their bespoke methods, freezing and thawing methodologies, the skill level of the embryologist, and the equipment they utilize to manage and store embryos. So, while success rates are important inputs to the selection process, it is more nuanced than the numbers on the page. Data points like clinic operations and failures of any kind are not on the yearly surveys. And when it comes to the marketing literature and data presented on websites, remember they can cherry-pick whatever presents their outcomes in the best possible light. One example of this is touting high pregnancy rates versus live birth rates, even though no one enters a fertility clinic because they love being pregnant without wanting a baby later. And don't forget, they can also refuse treatment for poor-prognosis patients.

There is a certain irony to the acronym ART, since many providers describe their approach as both an art and a science. While there is plenty of science to support some parts of the process, each clinic and provider still has their own method, even if you look at two clinics in the same city just blocks apart. The fertility industry changes constantly, with new options and equipment and analysis available all the time. From what medium is used in the petri dishes that grow your embryos to the environment in which the embryologists operate, or injection protocol, it's up to that provider to decide exactly how they practice. There is no universal consensus on the most correct and successful methods or best practices. This disparity is especially pronounced if you talk to practitioners in other countries, as there is not even agreement on whether to use fresh or frozen embryos when given the option.

Questions to ask a prospective reproductive endocrinologist

- What happens during an initial consultation?
- Will I have one doctor treating me throughout my cycle or will I see multiple doctors or a nurse during a cycle?
- Do you have weekend appointments?
- How often do you communicate with your patients? Through which channels?
- What is the timeline for my case?

- How long does an individual cycle last, and how many times will I need to go to the office? Will I need to take time off from work?

- What other testing do my partner and I need to do before treatment?

- Which treatment option is the best for me to try first?

- Will I have to take a lot of medications given my situation?

- Do you prefer PGT-A tested over non-PGT-A tested?

- Do you recommend ICSI?

- What is your stance on single-embryo transfer?

- What is the success rate of pregnancy and live birth with my situation?

- What specific method does the clinic use for freezing eggs and embryos?

- Do you prefer fresh or frozen eggs/embryos?

- How long after the transfer will I learn my results?

- How much will it cost including medications and the consult?

- Do you offer any IVF grants? Are there grants affiliated with your clinic?

- If I must pay out of pocket, does your clinic offer a payment plan or any cost benefits or work with a fertility insurer?

- If treatment is unsuccessful, what else can we try? Can we try any of these things in an earlier cycle?

- Is there anything I can do to improve my success before, during, and after?

- Are there any long-term side effects?
- Can you share database info for donors if needed?

You should always share a copy of your medical record and talk to at least two providers at different clinics to get their take on your diagnosis. Ask the aforementioned questions that feel relevant, share your thoughts, and if the treatment suggestions align, great. If not, get a third opinion to break the tie. Also know that in most clinics, nurses field most questions and aspects of treatment. So, you may see the reproductive endocrinologist at a first appointment, then not again until a retrieval or transfer.

WHEN TREATMENTS FAIL

Whether it happens because there are no viable eggs or sperm, a viable embryo fails to form, the embryo does not implant, or it implants and you miscarry—a failed treatment is devastating, and unfortunately, common. For most people, the devastation ranges from feeling broken or flawed or hopeless to stress-related to the high cost of each cycle or the inability to pay for another one. When a cycle fails, you'll have a debrief with your clinic. They'll do their best to explain why it may have failed and coordinate next steps. The age of eggs, embryo quality, sperm quality, chromosomal abnormalities, autoimmune disorders, existing health conditions, and lifestyle factors can all be possible causes.

If the sperm, egg, or embryo quality is the reason, and if they haven't done so already, most clinics will start by doing PGT-A to optimize the odds of success. You will be able to understand your options for future success—what additional tests and treatments might be helpful. They can tweak the process based on information learned in previous cycles. One unexpected benefit of fertility treatment is that you get much more visibility into what's happening with your body—and sometimes it can help find a diagnosis if you have an underlying condition that you don't even know about.

In cases where additional IVF cycles are unlikely to result in a successful pregnancy, or eggs or sperm aren't viable, you or your doctor may discuss when it might make sense to move on to egg, sperm, or embryo donation. If the problem is recurrent implantation failure or other physical issues making it difficult to carry a pregnancy, a gestational carrier or surrogate can be explored. If none of these are options, people who still wish to have a child may consider fostering or adoption—additional options that, like fertility treatment, offer hope to build a family but are not without significant cost, delay, and controversy as just like there is no "just relax" there is also no "just adopt." If you are trying to decide how or if to move forward, consider working with a fertility counselor or therapist. And lean on the people you love. You are never alone.

Fertility Treatment and Assisted Reproduction Wrap-Up

- An exact course of treatment depends on how long you've tried to conceive, your and your partner's ages, health, genetic, and fertility profiles, and what you can afford.

- The goal with fertility treatment is to start with less invasive, inexpensive treatments before moving on to IVF.

- Pending the diagnosis, your doctor may try medications like Clomid or change lifestyle factors before jumping into more invasive treatments.

- Using donor gametes or a surrogate or gestational carrier comes into play if IVF is unsuccessful.

- Interview at least two different reproductive

endocrinologists before choosing a clinic. Get a third opinion if the two don't agree.

- Navigating infertility is complicated, difficult, isolating, and emotional, so lean on friends and your partner, seek community with others in the trenches, or therapy if you need it.

After our second failed pregnancy, I asked if my ob-gyn if we should pursue assisted reproduction. She said no because the official guideline is to perform more rigorous testing and treatment after three consecutive miscarriages. At the time, I questioned whether it was the right next step to try again without intervention, but after a two month break, we got pregnant again—and this time, it stuck. To represent the lived experiences of fertility patients, I interviewed many friends and strangers who were kind enough to share their stories and provide feedback on all related content.

I'll leave you with this final thought. We are not forever defined as parents by what does or does not happen before conception or how our children enter the world. No matter what you do or how much you know, things do not always play out the way you'd like. Even with the depths of the knowledge I accumulated writing Bumpin', *my boys did not arrive the way I expected or hoped they would. But the only thing they see when they look at me now is their mom.*

GLOSSARY

ABBREVIATIONS YOU MAY ENCOUNTER ON YOUR FERTILITY JOURNEY

ART—assisted reproduction treatments

BBT—basal body temperature

CBT—cognitive behavioral therapy

D&C—dilation and curettage

DHEA—dehydroepiandrosterone (a fertility supplement used to treat diminished ovarian reserve)

DOR—diminished ovarian reserve

EDC—endocrine-disrupting chemicals

FAM—fertility-awareness method (also known as natural family planning)

FSH—follicle-stimulating hormone

HCG—human chorionic gonadotropin (the pregnancy hormone)

HPA—hypothalamic-pituitary-adrenal axis

IBD—inflammatory bowel disease

IBS—irritable bowel syndrome

ICI—intracervical insemination

ICSI—intracytoplasmic sperm injection

IUD—intrauterine device

IUI—intrauterine insemination

IVF—in vitro fertilization

LARC—long-acting contraceptive

LH—luteinizing hormone

LMP—last menstrual period

mtDNA—mitochondrial DNA

NIPT—noninvasive prenatal testing

OPK—ovulation-prediction kit

OTP—ovarian tissue preservation

PCOS—polycystic ovarian syndrome

PID—pelvic inflammatory disease

PRS—polygenic risk scores

SSRI—selective serotonin reuptake inhibitor

TSH—thyroid-stimulating hormone

TSS—toxic shock syndrome

TTC—trying to conceive

TWW—two-week wait

UTI—urinary tract infection

ACKNOWLEDGMENTS

Thank you to the readers of Bumpin' for inspiring this book. I love getting your notes and hope Fertility Rules provides the answers you seek.

A giant, heartfelt thanks to my agent Julia Eagleton at Janklow & Nesbit, for the riffs, edits, and steadfast support from our first conversation. I couldn't be more grateful for your friendship and look forward to many more literary adventures.

To my editorial team at Simon Element, Leah Miller, and Emma Taussig, thank you for understanding that this book needed to exist and for your pushes to whittle and make it better. Btw Emma, your knowledge of medical anthropology is astounding. Kate Davids, thank you for the early insights that helped it take shape. Thanks also to Patrick Sullivan, Lexy East, Laura Jarrett, Jessie McNiel, Elizabeth Breeden, Zoe Miller, and Erica Ferguson for the hard work behind the scenes to make this book.

To my medical dream team: Jane van Dis, thanks for going on another wild ride with me and believing in this project from the start. Christopher De Jonge, your infectious zeal for men's health changed the scope and focus of this book—let's hope it has our desired effect.

To my clinical experts: Michaela Burns, thank you for teaching me so much about human physiology. Liz Miracle, I am in awe of your ability to make pelvic health awesomely simple. And Aliza Marogy, you are a brilliant clinician and entrepreneur and a marvelous friend.

My eternal thanks to Kate Ryder for igniting my early passion for this topic, friendship, and relentlessly advocating for families. Thanks to Paxton Maeder-York for additions to the assisted reproduction content and for doing something about the lack of standardization in ART. Thanks Khaled Kteily, aka the Sperm King, for helping me understand how to better write for men and for making sperm testing and storage available for anyone who wants it. Dina Radenkovic, thanks for helping me see the future of fertility and actually building it. Carine Carmy, thanks for lending me Liz and shining a bright light on the physical side of women's health. Camilla Hermann and Michelle Stephens, thank you both for highlighting the often overlooked power of community. And Ellie Powers, your edits and feedback were incredible and invaluable. I look forward to returning the favor when you're ready.

I spoke to countless fertility experts while researching this book, including many that did so candidly on background. A special thanks to David Stern, Thilo Kleinschmidt, Natan Bar-Chama, Barb Colloran, Kurt Miller, Pasquale Patrizio, Atsushi Tanaka, Helen O'Neill, Hélène Guillaume, Dana McQueen, and Michael Eisenberg for sharing your perspective in explicit detail. Thanks also to Lawrence Wright for great intros.

To the ridiculously talented team of photographer Caitlin Mitchell and makeup artist Mary Irwin, thank you for the education, and for pulling me out of my postpartum haze with new headshots.

I am lucky to have rad friends that served as editors and soundboards, especially Megan Miller, Linda Avey, Kathy Chan, Susan Coelius Keplinger, Emily Goligoski, Talia Krohn, Lisa Forster, and Gesche Haas. To the womb—Chrissy Farr, Aike Ho, Alyssa Jaffe, and Deena Shakir—you keep me sane, entertained, inspired, and I cherish each of you and our crew. A special shout out to Chrissy for unwavering support from the proposal through pub day and the many rounds of edits. I can't wait for your turn. And Ryan Panchadsaram, you always have my back, and I'll always have yours. You are the bestest.

It takes a village to support working parents. Without Danielle

Sackett this book wouldn't be here—thank you thank you. My father, Jim Ziegler aka Pop, stepped in not once but twice to save our butts. We are so grateful for you, dad.

Reading Stephen King's book On Writing in college deeply affected me. I reflect on his advice to writers often, from reading a lot to keeping your writing simple. On the first point, I thank my mother, Gayle Ziegler, for raising a reader.

TJ and Dylan, by the time you read this, I hope you're not embarrassed that I'm your mom and understand that I write because I want the world to be better for you. You bring me joy I didn't realize was possible.

Nick, you endured hours of research ratholes over dinner and walks without a single complaint—again. You are a great dad, let me be my best and most true self, and are my partner in crime and in life. I love you so much.

BIBLIOGRAPHY

INTRODUCTION

Barratt, C. L. R., C. J. De Jonge, R. A. Anderson, M. L. Eisenberg, N. Garrido, S. Rautakallio Hokkanen, C. Krausz, S. Kimmins, M. K. O'Bryan, A. A. Pacey, et al. "A Global Approach to Addressing the Policy, Research and Social Challenges of Male Reproductive Health." *Human Reproduction Open* 2021, no. 1 (March 21, 2021): hoab009. https://doi.org/10.1093/hropen/hoab009.

Cleveland Clinic. "2019 Cleveland Clinic MENtion It Survey Results Overview." September 4, 2019. https://newsroom.clevelandclinic.org /wp-content/uploads/sites/4/2019/09/2019-Cleveland-Clinic-MEN tion-It-Survey-Results-Overview.pdf.

De Jonge, C., and C. L. R. Barratt. "The Present Crisis in Male Reproductive Health: An Urgent Need for a Political, Social, and Research Roadmap." *Andrology* 7, no. 6 (November 2019): 762–68. https://doi .org/10.1111/andr.12673.

Gleicher, N., V. A. Kushnir, and D. H. Barad. "Worldwide Decline of IVF Birth Rates and Its Probable Causes." *Human Reproduction Open* 2019, no. 3 (2019). https://doi.org/10.1093/hropen/hoz017.

Halpern, J. A., A. L. Darves-Bornoz, R. J. Fantus, M. K. Keeter, J. Wren, N. E. Bennett, and R. E. Brannigan. "Underutilization of Primary Medical Care Among Men Presenting for Fertility Evaluation." *F&S Reports* 1, no. 1 (June 1, 2020): 9–14. https://doi.org/10.1016/j.xfre.2020.04.001.

Johnson, M. H., S. B. Franklin, M. Cottingham, and N. Hopwood. "Why the Medical Research Council Refused Robert Edwards and Patrick Steptoe Support for Research on Human Conception in 1971." *Human Reproduction* 25, no. 9 (September 1, 2010): 2157–74. https:// doi.org/10.1093/humrep/deq155.

Kudesia, R., E. Chernyak, and B. McAvey. "Low Fertility Awareness in United States Reproductive-Aged Women and Medical Trainees: Creation and Validation of the Fertility & Infertility Treatment Knowledge Score (FIT-KS)." *Fertility and Sterility* 108, no. 4 (October 1, 2017): 711–17. https://doi.org/10.1016/j.fertnstert.2017.07.1158.

Latif, T., T. Kold Jensen, J. Mehlsen, S. A. Holmboe, L. Brinth, K. Pors, S. O. Skouby, N. Jørgensen, and R. Lindahl-Jacobsen. "Semen Quality as a Predictor of Subsequent Morbidity: A Danish Cohort Study of 4,712 Men with Long-Term Follow-up." *American Journal of Epidemiology* 186, no. 8 (October 15, 2017): 910–17. https://doi.org/10.1093/aje/kwx067.

Levine, H., N. Jørgensen, A. Martino-Andrade, J. Mendiola, D. Weksler-Derri, I. Mindlis, R. Pinotti, and S. H. Swan. "Temporal Trends in Count: A Systematic Review and Meta-Regression Analysis." *Human Reproduction Update* 23, no. 6 (November–December 2017): 646–59. https://doi.org/10.1093/humupd/dmx022.

National Center for Health Statistics. "Infertility." Centers for Disease Control and Prevention. Accessed September 13, 2022. https://www.cdc.gov/nchs/fastats/infertility.htm.

National Institutes of Health. "How Common Is Infertility?" US Department of Health and Human Services. Accessed September 13, 2022. https://www.nichd.nih.gov/health/topics/infertility/conditioninfo/common.

———. "Educating Teenagers about Sex in the United States." Centers for Disease Control and Prevention. Accessed July 27, 2022. https://www.cdc.gov/nchs/products/databriefs/db44.htm.

Scott, I. A., and C. Crock. "Diagnostic Error: Incidence, Impacts, Causes and Preventive Strategies." *Medical Journal of Australia* 213, no. 7 (October 2020): 302–05. https://doi.org/10.5694/mja2.50771.

Steiner, A. Z., D. Pritchard D, and F. Z. Stanczyk. "Association Between Biomarkers of Ovarian Reserve and Infertility Among Older Women of Reproductive Age." *Journal of the American Medical Association* 318, no. 14 (October 10, 2017): 1367–76. http://doi.org/10.1001/jama.2017.14588.

Tseng, C.-H. "The Effect of Metformin on Male Reproductive Function and Prostate: An Updated Review." *World Journal of Men's Health* 40, no. 1 (January 2022): 11–29. https://doi.org/10.5534/wjmh.210001.

Walsh, T. J., M. S. Croughan, M. Schembri, J. M. Chan, and P. J. Turek. "Increased Risk of Testicular Germ Cell Cancer Among Infertile Men." *Archives of Internal Medicine* 169, no. 4 (February 23, 2009): 351–56. https://doi.org/10.1001/archinternmed.2008.562.

CHAPTER 1: THE MENSTRUAL CYCLE

Abdelmonem, A., S. M. Rasheed, and A. Sh. Mohamed. "Bee-Honey and Yogurt: A Novel Mixture for Treating Patients with Vulvovaginal Candidiasis during Pregnancy." *Archives of Gynecology and Obstetrics* 286, no. 1 (February 8, 2012): 109–14. https://doi.org/10.1007/s00404-012-2242-5.

ActionAid. "1 in 4 UK Women Don't Understand Their Menstrual Cycle." May 23, 2017. https://www.actionaid.org.uk/blog/news/2017/05/24/1-in-4-uk-women-dont-understand-their-menstrual-cycle.

Barth, C., C. Steele, K. Mueller, V. P. Pekkas, K. Arélin, A. Pampel, I. Burmann, J. Kratzsch, A. Villringer, and J. Sacher. "*In-vivo* Dynamics of the Human Hippocampus across the Menstrual Cycle." *Scientific Reports* 6 (2016): article 32833. https://doi.org/10.1038/srep32833.

Boutot, Meagan. "Toxic Shock Syndrome (TSS) and Menstrual Products: A Short History." Clue. April 22, 2019. https://helloclue.com/articles/cycle-a-z/toxic-shock-syndrome-and-menstrual-products-a-short-history.

Bull, J. R., S. P. Rowland, E. B. Scherwitzl, R. Scherwitzl, K. G. Danielsson, and J. Harper. "Real-World Menstrual Cycle Characteristics of More Than 600,000 Menstrual Cycles," *Digital Medicine* 2, (2019): article 83. https://doi.org/10.1038/s41746-019-0152-7.

Chalabi, Mona. "How Many Women Don't Use Tampons?" FiveThirtyEight. October 1, 2015. https://fivethirtyeight.com/features/how-many-women-dont-use-tampons/.

Clearblue. "Accuracy of Recollection of Last Menstrual Period." Accessed September 13, 2022. https://es.clearblue.com/sites/default/files/HCP_Publications/Articles-Pregnancy/Accuracy_of_recollection_of_Last_Menstrual_Period.pdf.

DeVito, M. J., and A. Schecter. "Exposure Assessment to Dioxins from the Use of Tampons and Diapers." *Environmental Health Perspectives* 110, no. 1 (January 2002): 23–28. https://doi.org/10.1289/ehp.0211023.

Fitzgerald, M., L. Pritschet, T. Santander, S. T. Grafton, and E. G. Jacobs. "Cerebellar Network Organization across the Human Menstrual Cycle," *Scientific Reports* 10 (2020): article 20732. https://doi.org/10.1038/s41598-020-77779-4.

Grewal, K., Y. S. Lee, A. Smith, J. J. Brosens, T. Bourne, M. Al-Memar, S. Kundu, D. MacIntyre, and P. R. Bennett. "Chromosomally Normal Miscarriage Is Associated with Vaginal Dysbiosis and Local Inflammation." *BMC Medicine* 20 (2022): article 38. https://doi.org/10.1186/s12916-021-02227-7.

Hartmann, K. E., C. Fonnesbeck, T. Surawicz, S. Krishnaswami, J. C. Andrews, J. E. Wilson, D. Velez-Edwards, S. Kugley, and N. A. Santhe. "Management of Uterine Fibroids." *Agency for Healthcare Research and Quality* 195 (December 2017). https://www.ncbi.nlm.nih.gov /books/NBK537747.

Hudson, N. "The Missed Disease? Endometriosis as an Example of 'Undone Science.'" *Reproductive Biomedicine & Society Online* 14 (August 13, 2021): 20–27. https://doi.org/10.1016/j.rbms.2021.07.003.

Koumans, E. H., M. Sternberg, C. Bruce, G. McQuillan, J. Kendrick, M. Sutton, and L. E. Markowitz. "The Prevalence of Bacterial Vaginosis in the United States, 2001–2004; Associations with Symptoms, Sexual Behaviors, and Reproductive Health." *Sexually Transmitted Diseases* 34, no. 11 (November 2007): 864–69. https://doi.org/10.1097 /OLQ.0b013e318074e565.

Monis, C. N. and M. Tetrokalashvili. "Menstrual Cycle Proliferative and Follicular Phase." *StatPearls* (January 2022). https://www.ncbi.nlm .nih.gov/books/NBK542229/.

Nikokavoura, E. A., K. L. Johnston, J. Broom, W. L. Wrieden, and C. Rolland. "Weight Loss for Women with and without Polycystic Ovary Syndrome Following a Very Low-Calorie Diet in a Community-Based Setting with Trained Facilitators for 12 weeks." *Diabetes, Metabolic Syndrome and Obesity: Targets and Therapy* 8 (October 14, 2015): 495–503, https://doi.org/10.2147/DMSO.S85134.

Practice Committee of the American Society for Reproductive Medicine. "Endometriosis and Infertility: A Committee Opinion," *ASRM* 98, no. 3 (September 1, 2012): 591–98. https://doi.org/10.1016/j .fertnstert.2012.05.031.

Ravel, J., G. Pawel, Z. Zaid, and L. J. Forney. "Vaginal Microbiome of Reproductive-Age Women." *PNAS* 108, supp. 1 (June 3, 2010): 4680–87. https://doi.org/10.1073/pnas.1002611107.

Riazi, H., M. Ghazanfarpour, M. Taebi, and S. Abdolahian. "Effect of Vitamin D on the Vaginal Health of Menopausal Women: A Systematic Review." *Journal of Menopausal Medicine* 25, no. 3 (December 2019): 109–16. https://doi.org/10.6118/jmm.19194.

Siebert, Valerie. "Nearly Half of Women Have Experienced 'Period Shaming.'" *New York Post.* January 3, 2018. https://nypost.com/2018/01/03 /nearly-half-of-women-have-experienced-period-shaming.

Stanford, J. B., S. K. Willis, E. E. Hatch, K. J. Rothman, and L. A. Wise. "Fecundability in Relation to Use of Mobile Computing Apps to Track the Menstrual Cycle," *Human Reproduction* 35,

no. 10 (October 2020): 2245–52. https://doi.org/10.1093/humrep
/deaa176.

US Food and Drug Administration. "The Facts on Tampons—and How to Use
Them Safely." FDA. Accessed September 13, 2022. https://www.fda.gov
/consumers/consumer-updates/facts-tampons-and-how-use-them-safely.

van de Wijgert, J. H. H. M. "The Vaginal Microbiome and Sexually
Transmitted Infections Are Interlinked: Consequences for Treatment
and Prevention." *PLoS Med* 14, no. 12 (December 27, 2017):
e1002478. https://doi.org/10.1371/journal.pmed.1002478.

Witkin, S.S. and I. M. Linhares. "Why Do Lactobacilli Dominate the Human
Vaginal Microbiota?" *BJOG* 124, no. 4 (November 7, 2016): 606–11.
https://doi.org/10.1111/1471-0528.14390.

CHAPTER 2: EGGS

Balk, J., J. Catov, B. Horn, K. Gecsi, and A. Wakim. "The Relationship
Between Perceived Stress, Acupuncture, and Pregnancy Rates among
IVF Patients: A Pilot Study." *Complementary Therapies in Clinical
Practice* 16, no. 3 (August 2010): 154–57. https://doi.org/10.1016/j
.ctcp.2009.11.004.

Ben-Meir, A., E. Burstein, A. Borrego-Alvarez, J. Chong, E. Wong, T.
Yavorska, T. Naranian, M. Chi, Y. Wang, Y. Bentov, et al. "Coenzyme
Q10 Restores Oocyte Mitochondrial Function and Fertility during
Reproductive Aging." *Aging Cell* 14, no. 5 (October 2015): 887–95.
https://doi.org/10.1111/acel.12368.

Cascante, S. D., J. K. Blakemore, S. DeVore, B. Hodes-Wertz, M. E. Fino,
A. S. Berkeley, C. M. Parra, C. McCaffrey, and J. A. Grifo. "Fifteen
Years of Autologous Oocyte Thaw Outcomes from a Large University-
Based Fertility Center." *Fertility and Sterility* 118, no.1 (July 1, 2022):
158–166. https://doi.org/10.1016/j.fertnstert.2022.04.013

"Female Age-Related Fertility Decline." American College of Obstetricians
and Gynecologists Clinical. March 2014, reaffirmed 2022. https://
www.acog.org/clinical/clinical-guidance/committee-opinion
/articles/2014/03/female-age-related-fertility-decline.

Fouks, Y., A. Penzias, W. Neuhausser, D. Vaughan, and D. Sakkas. "A
Diagnosis of Diminished Ovarian Reserve Does Not Impact Embryo
Aneuploidy or Live Birth Rates Compared to Patients with Normal
Ovarian Reserve," *Fertility and Sterility* 118, no. 3 (September 1, 2022):
504–12. https://doi.org/10.1016/j.fertnstert.2022.06.008.

Fragouli, E., K. Spath, S. Alfarawati, F. Kaper, A. Craig, C-E. Michel, F.

Kokocinski, J. Cohen, S. Munne, and D. Wells. "Altered Levels of Mitochondrial DNA Are Associated with Female Age, Aneuploidy, and Provide an Independent Measure of Embryonic Implantation Potential," *PLOS Genetics* 11, no. 6 (June 3, 2015). https://doi.org/10.1371/journal.pgen.1005241.

Herbert, M., D. Kalleas, D. Cooney, M. Lamb, and L. Lister. "Meiosis and Maternal Aging: Insights from Aneuploid Oocytes and Trisomy Births." *Cold Spring Harbor Perspectives in Biology* 7, no. 4 (2015). https://doi.org/10.1101/cshperspect.a017970.

Leridon, H. "Can Assisted Reproduction Technology Compensate for the Natural Decline in Fertility with Age? A Model Assessment." *Human Reproduction* 19, no. 7 (July 1, 2004): 1548–53. https://doi.org/10.1093/humrep/deh304.

So, C., K. Menelaou, J. Uraji, K. Harasimov, A. M. Steyer, K. B. Seres, J. Bucevičius, G. Lukinavičius, W. Möbius, C. Sibold, et al. "Mechanism of Spindle Pole Organization and Instability in Human Oocytes." *Science* 375, no. 6581 (February 11, 2022). https://doi.org/10.1126/science.abj3944.

Steiner, A. Z., D. Pritchard, F. Z. Stanczyk, J. S. Kesner, J. W. Meadows, A. H. Herring, and D. D. Baird. "Association Between Biomarkers of Ovarian Reserve and Infertility Among Older Women of Reproductive Age." *JAMA* 318, no. 14 (October 10, 2017): 1367–76. https://doi.org/10.1001/jama.2017.14588.

Thomas, C., T. Cavazza, and M. Schuh. "Aneuploidy in Human Eggs: Contributions of the Meiotic Spindle." *Biochemical Society Transactions* 49, no. 1 (February 2021): 107–18. https://doi.org/10.1042/BST20200043.

Zheng, C. H., M. M. Zhang, G. Y. Huang, and W. Wang. "The Role of Acupuncture in Assisted Reproductive Technology," *Evidence-Based Complementary and Alternative Medicine* 2012 (July 2, 2012). https://doi.org/10.1155/2012/543924.

CHAPTER 3: SPERM

Al Shareef, S., S. B. Gokarakonda, R. Marwaha. "Anabolic Steroid Use Disorder." *StatPearls* (2022). https://www.ncbi.nlm.nih.gov/books/NBK538174/.

Alwaal, A., B. N. Breyer, and T. F. Lue. "Normal Male Sexual Function: Emphasis on Orgasm and Ejaculation." *Fertility and Sterility* 104, no. 5 (November 1, 2015): 1051–60. https://doi.org/10.1016/j.fertnstert.2015.08.033.

Barratt, C., C. J. De Jonge, R. A. Anderson, M. L. Eisenberg, N. Garrido, S.

Rautakallio Hokkanen, C. Krausz, S. Kimmins, M. K. O'Bryan, A. A. Pacey, et al. "A Global Approach to Addressing the Policy, Research and Social Challenges of Male Reproductive Health." *Human Reproduction Open* 2021, no. 1 (2021). https://doi.org/10.1093/hropen/hoab009.

Boland, M. J., J. L. Hazen, K. L. Nazor, A. R. Rodriguez, G. Martin, S. Kupriyanov, and K. K. Baldwin. "Generation of Mice Derived from Induced Pluripotent Stem Cells." *Journal of Visualized Experiments* 69 (November 29, 2012): e4003, https://doi.org/10.3791/4003.

Brannigan, R., and L. Lipshultz. "Sperm Transport and Capacitation." *Global Library of Women's Medicine's Welfare of Women Global Health Programme* (2008). https://doi.org/10.3843/GLOWM.10316.

D'Angelo, S., and R. Meccariello. "Microplastics: A Threat for Male Fertility." *International Journal of Environmental Research and Public Health* 18, no. 5 (March 1, 2021): 2392. https://doi.org/10.3390/ijerph18052392.

Jónsson, H., P. Sulem, B. Kehr, S. Kristmundsdottir, F. Zink, E. Hjartarson, M. T. Hardarson, K. E. Hjorleifsson, H. P. Eggertsson, S. A. Gudjonsson, et al. "Parental Influence on Human Germline *De Novo* Mutations in 1,548 Trios from Iceland." *Nature* 549 (September 20, 2017): 519–22. https://doi.org/10.1038/nature24018.

Jung, A., P. Strauss, H.-J. Lindner, and H.C. Schuppe. "Influence of Heating Car Seats on Scrotal Temperature." *Fertility and Sterility* 90, no. 2 (August 1, 2008): 335–39. https://doi.org/10.1016/j.fertnstert.2007.06.053.

Lea, R. G., A. Byers, R. Sumner, S. M. Rhind, Z. Shang, S. L. Freeman, R. Moxon, H. M. Richardson, M. Green, J. Craigon, and G. C. W. England. "Environmental Chemicals Impact Dog Semen Quality In Vitro and May Be Associated with a Temporal Decline in Sperm Motility and Increased Cryptorchidism." *Scientific Reports* 6 (2016): article 31281. https://doi.org/10.1038/srep31281.

Levitas E., E. Lunenfeld, N. Weisz, M. Friger, and G. Potashnik. "Relationship Between Age and Semen Parameters in Men with Normal Sperm Concentration: Analysis of 6022 Semen Samples." *Andrologia* 39, no. 2 (April 5, 2007): 45–50. https://doi.org/10.1111/j.1439-0272.2007.00761.x.

Mathieu, C., R. Ecochard, V. Bied, J. Lornage, and J. C. Czyba. "Andrology: Cumulative Conception Rate Following Intrauterine Artificial Insemination with Husband's Spermatozoa: Influence of Husband's Age." *Human reproduction* 10, no. 5 (May 1, 1995): 1090–97. https://doi.org/10.1093/oxfordjournals.humrep.a136100.

Mínguez-Alarcón, L., A. Gaskins, Y.H. Chiu, C. Messerlian, P. L. Williams, J.

B. Ford, I. Souter, R. Hauser, and J. E. Chavarro. "Type of Underwear Worn and Markers of Testicular Function Among Men Attending a Fertility Center." *Human Reproduction* 33, no. 9 (September 2018): 1749–56. https://doi.org/10.1093/humrep/dey259.

Nikolopoulos, I., W. Osman, Z. Haoula, K. Jayaprakasan, and W. Atiomo. "Scrotal Cooling and Its Benefits to Male Fertility: A Systematic Review." *Journal of Obstetrics and Gynaecology* 33, no. 4 (2013): 338–42. https://doi.org/10.3109/01443615.2012.758088.

Phillips, N., L. Taylor, and G. Bachmann. "Maternal, Infant and Childhood Risks Associated with Advanced Paternal Age: The Need for Comprehensive Counseling for Men." *Maturitas* 125 (July 1, 2019): 81–84. https://doi.org/10.1016/j.maturitas.2019.03.020.

Pino, V., A. Sanz, N. Valdés, J. Crosby, and A. Mackenna. "The Effects of Aging on Semen Parameters and Sperm DNA Fragmentation." *JBRA Assisted Reproduction* 24, no. 1 (January 30, 2020): 82–86. https://doi.org/10.5935/1518-0557.20190058.

Poppick, Laura. "The Long, Winding Tale of Sperm Science." *Smithsonian Magazine.* June 7, 2017. https://www.smithsonianmag.com/science-nature/scientists-finally-unravel-mysteries-sperm-180963578/.

Sales, K., R. Vasudeva, M. E. Dickinson, J. L. Godwin, A. J. Lumley, Ł. Michalczyk, L. Hebberecht, P. Thomas, A. Franco, and M. J. G. Gage. "Experimental Heatwaves Compromise Sperm Function and Cause Transgenerational Damage in a Model Insect." *Nature Communications* 9 (2018): article 4771. https://doi.org/10.1038/s41467-018-07273-z.

Stahl, Michael. "The Legend of Horst Schultz, the World's Most Famous Long-Distance Ejaculator." *Mel.* Accessed September 13, 2022. https://melmagazine.com/en-us/story/biggest-cumshot-horst-schultz-long-distance-ejaculation.

Wensink, M. J., Y. Lu, L. Tian, G. Shaw, S. Rizzi, T. K. Jensen, E. R. Mathiesen, N. E. Shakkebæk, R. Lindahl-Jacobsen, and M. L. Eisenberg. "Preconception Antidiabetic Drugs in Men and Birth Defects in Offspring: A Nationwide Cohort Study." *Annals of Internal Medicine* (May 2022). https://doi.org/10.7326/M21-4389.

CHAPTER 4: HORMONES

Allen, W. M., and G. W. Corner. "Physiology of the Corpus Luteum." *American Journal of Physiology* 88, no. 2 (March 1929): 340–46. https://doi.org/10.1152/ajplegacy.1929.88.2.340.

Gentry-Maharaj, A., C. Karpinskyj, C. Glazer, M. Burnell, A. Ryan,

L. Fraser, A. Lanceley, I. Jacobs, M. S. Hunter, and U. Menon. "Use and Perceived Efficacy of Complementary and Alternative Medicines after Discontinuation of Hormone Therapy." *Menopause* 22, no. 4 (April 22, 2015): 384–90. https://doi.org/10.1097/GME.0000000000000330.

Lopresti, A. L., P. D. Drummond, and S. J. Smith. "A Randomized, Double-Blind, Placebo-Controlled, Crossover Study Examining the Hormonal and Vitality Effects of Ashwagandha (*Withania somnifera*) in Aging, Overweight Males." *American Journal of Men's Health* 13, no. 2 (March 10, 2019). https://doi.org/10.1177/1557988319835985.

Melado, L., B. Lawrenz, J. Sibal, E. Abu, C. Coughlan, A. T. Navarro, and H. M. Fatemi. "Anti-müllerian Hormone during Natural Cycle Presents Significant Intra and Intercycle Variations When Measured with Fully Automated Assay." *Frontiers in Endocrinology* (November 27, 2018). https://doi.org/10.3389/fendo.2018.00686.

Pilz, S., S. Frisch, H. Koertke, J. Kuhn, J. Dreier, B. Obermayer-Pietsch, E. Wehr, and A. Zittermann. "Effect of Vitamin D Supplementation on Testosterone Levels in Men." *Hormone and Metabolic Research* 43, no. 3 (2011): 223–25. https://doi.org/10.1055/s-0030-1269854.

Vaamonde, D., M. E. Da Silva-Grigoletto, J. M. García-Manso, N. Barrera, and R. Vaamonde-Lemos. "Physically Active Men Show Better Semen Parameters and Hormone Values than Sedentary Men." *European Journal of Applied Physiology* 112, no. 9 (January 11, 2012): 3267–73. https://doi.org/10.1007/s00421-011-2304-6.

Van Iten, Brendan. "Edgar Allen and Edward A. Doisy's Extraction of Estrogen from Ovarian Follicles, (1923)." *Embryo Project Encyclopedia*. March 2, 2017. ISSN: 1940–5030. http://embryo.asu.edu/handle/10776/11433.

CHAPTER 5: BIRTH CONTROL

Agboola, S., and J. Kvedar. "Telemedicine and Patient Safety." Agency for Healthcare Research and Quality. September 16, 2016. https://psnet.ahrq.gov/perspective/telemedicine-and-patient-safety.

Allen, R., and B. M. O'Brien. "Uses of Misoprostol in Obstetrics and Gynecology." *Reviews in Obstetrics & Gynecology* 2, no. 3 (September 2009): 159–68. https://www.ncbi.nlm.nih.gov/pmc/articles/PMC2760893/pdf/RIOG002003_0159.pdf.

"Challenges to Choice." United Nations Population Fund. Accessed September 13, 2022. https://www.unfpa.org/swp2022/challenges.

Chang, Z., W. Qin, H. Zheng, K. Schlegg, L. Han, X. Liu, Z. Wang, H. McSqiggin, H. Peng, S. Yuan, et al. "Triptonide Is a Reversible

Non-Hormonal Male Contraceptive Agent in Mice and Non-Human Primates." *Nature Communications* 12 (February 23, 2021): article 1253. https://doi.org/10.1038/s41467-021-21517-5.

Cleveland Clinic. "Vasectomy Reversal: Facts You Need to Know." September 13, 2022. https://health.clevelandclinic.org/how-reversible-are-vasectomies/.

Clinicaltrials.gov. "Study of Daily Application of Nestorone® (NES) and Testosterone (T) Combination Gel for Male Contraception." US National Library of Medicine. Accessed September 13, 2022. https://clinicaltrials.gov/ct2/show/NCT03452111.

"Crocodile or Elephant Dung." Museum of Contraception and Abortion. Accessed September 13, 2022. https://muvs.org/en/contraception/barriers/crocodile-or-elephant-dung-id2519/.

Farrow, A., M. G. R. Hull, K. Northstone, H. Taylor, W. C. L. Ford, and J. Golding. "Prolonged Use of Oral Contraception Before a Planned Pregnancy Is Associated with a Decreased Risk of Delayed Conception." *Human Reproduction* 17, no. 10 (October 2002): 2754–61. https://doi.org/10.1093/humrep/17.10.2754.

Girum, T., and A. Wasie. "Return of Fertility after Discontinuation of Contraception: A Systematic Review and Meta-Analysis." *Contraception and Reproductive Medicine* 3 (July 23, 2018): article 9. https://doi.org/10.1186/s40834-018-0064-y.

Glasier, A.F., R. Anakwe, D. Everington, C. W. Martin, Z. van der Spuy, L. Cheng, P. C. Ho, and R. A. Anderson. "Would Women Trust Their Partners to Use a Male Pill?" *Human Reproduction* 15, no. 3 (March 1, 2000): 646–49. https://doi.org/10.1093/humrep/15.3.646.

Grossman, D., K. White, K. Hopkins, J. Amastae, M. Shedlin, and J. E. Potter. "Contraindications to Combined Oral Contraceptives among Over-the-Counter Compared with Prescription Users." *Obstetrics & Gynecology* 117, no. 3 (March 2011): 558–65. https://doi.org/10.1097/AOG.0b013e31820b0244.

Jain, T., E. Schwarz, and A. Mehrotra. "A Study of Telecontraception." *New England Journal of Medicine* 381, no. 13 (September 26, 2019): 1287–88. https://doi.org/10.1056/NEJMc1907545.

Kirubarajan, A., X. Li, M. Yau, C. Yu, T. Got, Q. Li, E. Huszti, S. Leung, N. Thangavelu, and M. Sobel. "Awareness, Knowledge, and Misconceptions of Adolescents and Young People Regarding Long-Acting Reversible Contraceptives: A Systematic Review and Meta-Analysis." *Fertility and Sterility* 118, no. 1 (July 1, 2022): 168–79. https://doi.org/10.1016/j.fertnstert.2022.03.013.

Martin, C. W., R. A. Anderson, L. Cheng, P. C. Ho, Z. van der Spuy, K. B.

Smith, A. F. Glasier, D. Everington, and D. T. Baird. "Potential Impact of Hormonal Male Contraception: Cross-Cultural Implications for Development of Novel Preparations." *Human Reproduction* 15, no. 3 (March 1, 2000): 637–45. https://doi.org/10.1093/humrep/15.3.637.

Mikkelsen, E. M., A. H. Riis, L. A. Wise, E. E. Hatch, K. J. Rothman, and H. T. Sørensen. "Pre-Gravid Oral Contraceptive Use and Time to Pregnancy: A Danish Prospective Cohort Study." *Human Reproduction* 28, no. 5 (May 2013): 1398–405. https://doi.org/10.1093/humrep/det023.

National Health Service. "Risks: Abortion." Accessed September 13, 2022. https://www.nhs.uk/conditions/abortion/risks/.

Planned Parenthood. "Birth Control." Accessed September 13, 2022. https://www.plannedparenthood.org/learn/birth-control.

———. "Abortion." Accessed September 13, 2022. https://www.plannedparenthood.org/learn/abortion.

Quarini, C. A. "History of Contraception." *Women's Health Medicine* 2, no. 5 (September 2005): 28–30. https://doi.org/10.1383/wohm.2005.2.5.28.

Robinson, J. A., and A. E. Burke. "Obesity and Hormonal Contraceptive Efficacy." *Women's Health* 9, no. 5 (September 2013): 453–66. https://doi.org/10.2217/whe.13.41.

"Why Don't We Have a Male Birth Control Pill Yet?" Episode 268, transcript. Science History Institute. April 20, 2021. https://www.sciencehistory.org/distillations/podcast/why-dont-we-have-a-male-birth-control-pill-yet#transcript.

Worly, B. L., T. L. Gur, and J. Schaffir. "The Relationship Between Progestin Hormonal Contraception and Depression: A Systematic Review." *Contraception* 97, no. 6 (June 1, 2018): 478–89. https://doi.org/10.1016/j.contraception.2018.01.010.

Yland, J. J., K. A. Bresnick, E. E. Hatch, A. K. Wesselink, E. M. Mikkelsen, K. J. Rothman, H. T. Sørensen, K. F. Huybrechts, and L. A. Wise. "Pregravid Contraceptive Use and Fecundability: Prospective Cohort Study." *BMJ* 2020, no. 371 (September 18, 2020): 3966. https://doi.org/10.1136/bmj.m3966.

CHAPTER 6: NUTRITION AND GUT HEALTH

Adams, K., M. Kohlmeier, and S. Zeisel. "Nutrition Education in U.S. Medical Schools: Latest Update of a National Survey." *Academic Medicine* 85, no. 9 (September 2010): 1537–42. https://doi.org/10.1097/ACM.0b013e3181eab71b.

Aoun, A., V. El Khoury, and R. Malakieh. "Can Nutrition Help in the Treatment of Infertility?" *Preventive Nutrition and Food Science* 26, no. 2 (June 30, 2021): 109–20. https://doi.org/10.3746/pnf.2021.26.2.109.

Baldridge, A. S., M. D. Huffman, F. Taylor, D. Xavier, B. Bright, L. V. Van Horn, B. Neal, and E. Dunford. "The Healthfulness of the US Packaged Food and Beverage Supply: A Cross-Sectional Study." *Nutrients* 11, no. 8 (July 24, 2019): 1704. https://doi.org/10.3390/nu11081704.

Blusztajn, J. K., and T. J. Mellott. "Neuroprotective Actions of Perinatal Choline Nutrition." *Clinical Chemistry and Laboratory Medicine* 51, no. 3 (January 3, 2013): 591–99. https://doi.org/10.1515/cclm-2012-0635.

Bowers, K., D. K. Tobias, E. Yeung, F. B. Hu, and C. Zhang. "A Prospective Study of Prepregnancy Dietary Fat Intake and Risk of Gestational Diabetes." *American Journal of Clinical Nutrition* 95, no. 2 (February 2012): 446–53. https://doi.org/10.3945/ajcn.111.026294.

Chavarro, J. E., J. W. Rich-Edwards, B. Rosner, and W. C. Willett. "A Prospective Study of Dairy Foods Intake and Anovulatory Infertility." *Human Reproduction* 22, no. 5 (May 1, 2007): 1340–47. https://doi.org/10.1093/humrep/dem019.

Chavarro, J. E., J. W. Rich-Edwards, B. A. Rosner, and W. Willett. "Dietary Fatty Acid Intakes and the Risk of Ovulatory Infertility." *American Journal of Clinical Nutrition* 85, no. 1 (January 2007): 231–37. https://doi.org/10.1093/ajcn/85.1.231.

Cito, G., A. Cocci, E. Micelli, A. Gabutti, G. I. Russo, M. E. Coccia, G. Franco, S. Serni, M. Carini, and A. Natali. "Vitamin D and Male Fertility: An Updated Review." *World Journal of Men's Health* 38, no. 2 (April 2020): 164–77. https://doi.org/10.5534/wjmh.190057.

Frisch, R. "The Right Weight: Body Fat, Menarche and Ovulation." *Baillière's Clinical Obstetrics and Gynaecology*, 4, no. 3 (September 1990): 419–39. https://doi.org/10.1016/S0950-3552(05)80302-5.

Gacesa, R., A. Kurilshikov, A. Vich Vila, T. Sinha, M. A. Y. Klaassen, L. A. Bolte, S. Andreu-Sánchez, L. Chen, V. Collij, S. Hu, et al. "Environmental Factors Shaping the Gut Microbiome in a Dutch Population." *Nature* 604, no. 7905 (April 14, 2022): 732–39. https://doi.org/10.1038/s41586-022-04567-7.

Gaskins, A. J., J. W. Rich-Edwards, P. L. Williams, T. L. Toth, S. A. Missmer, and J. E. Chavarro. "Prepregnancy Low to Moderate Alcohol Intake Is Not Associated with Risk of Spontaneous Abortion or Stillbirth." *Journal of Nutrition* 146, no. 4 (April 2016): 799–805. https://doi.org/10.3945/jn.115.226423.

Gaskins, A. J., T. L. Toth, and J. E. Chavarro. "Prepregnancy Nutrition and Early Pregnancy Outcomes." *Current Nutrition Reports* 4, no. 3 (September 2015): 265–72. https://doi.org/10.1007 /s13668-015-0127-5.

Gaskins A., Y.H. Chiu, P. Williams, R. Hauser, J. E. Chavarro. "Maternal Whole Grain Intake and Outcomes of In Vitro Fertilization." *Fertility and Sterility* 105, no. 6 (June 1, 2016): 1503–10. https://doi .org/10.1016/j.fertnstert.2016.02.015.

Ge, L., B. Sadeghirad, G. D. C. Ball, B. R. da Costa, C. L. Hitchcock, A. Svendrovski, R. Kiflen, K Quadri, H. Ywon, M. Karamouzian, T. Adams-Webber, et al. "Comparison of Dietary Macronutrient Patterns of 14 Popular Named Dietary Programmes for Weight and Cardiovascular Risk Factor Reduction in Adults: Systematic Review and Network Meta-Analysis of Randomised Trials." *BMJ* 2020, no. 369 (2020): m696. https://doi.org/10.1136/bmj.m696.

Guasch-Ferré, M., Y. Li, W. C. Willett, Q. Sun, L. Sampson, J. Salas-Salvadó, M. A. Martínez-González, M. J. Stampfer,Hu FB, *Journal of American College of Cardiology* 79, no. 2 (January 18, 2022): 101–12. https://doi .org/10.1016/j.jacc.2021.10.041.

Guo, D., M. Xu, Q. Zhou, C. Wu, R. Ju, and J. Dai. "Is Low Body Mass Index a Risk Factor for Semen Quality? A PRISMA-Compliant Meta-Analysis." *Medicine* 98, no. 32 (August 2019): e16677. https://doi .org/10.1097/MD.0000000000016677.

Halldorsson, T. I., M. Strøm, S. B. Petersen, and S. F. Olsen. "Intake of Artificially Sweetened Soft Drinks and Risk of Preterm Delivery: A Prospective Cohort Study in 59,334 Danish Pregnant Women." *American Journal of Clinical Nutrition* 92, no. 3 (September 2010): 626–33. https://doi.org/10.3945/ajcn.2009.28968.

Halpern, G., D. P. Braga, A. S. Setti, R. C. Figueria, A. Iaconelli, and E. Borges. "Artificial Sweeteners: Do They Bear an Infertility Risk?" *Fertility and Sterility* 106, no. 3, supplement (September 1, 2016): E263. https://doi.org/10.1016/j.fertnstert.2016.07.759.

Hargrove, J. L. "History of the Calorie in Nutrition." *Journal of Nutrition* 136, no. 12 (December 2006): 2957–61. https://doi.org/10.1093 /jn/136.12.2957.

Hatch, E. E., A. K. Wesselink, K. A. Hahn, J. J. Michiel, E. M. Mikkelsen, H. T. Sorensen, K. J. Rothman, and L. A.Wise. "Intake of Sugar-Sweetened Beverages and Fecundability in a North American Preconception Cohort." *Epidemiology* 29, no. 3 (May 2018): 369–78. https://doi.org/10.1097/EDE.0000000000000812.

Himanshu, V. and D. Roshan. "By Product Type (Better-for-You, Meal Replacement, Weight Loss Supplement, Green Tea, and Low-Calorie Sweeteners) and Sales Channel (Hypermarket/Supermarket, Specialty Stores, Pharmacies, Online Channels, and Others): Global Opportunity Analysis and Industry Forecast, 2021–2027," in *Weight Loss and Weight Management Diet Market.* Allied Market Research. May 2021. https://www.alliedmarketresearch.com/weight-loss-management-diet-market.

Juul, F., N. Parekh, E. Martinez-Steele, C. A. Monteiro, and V. W. Chang. "Ultra-Processed Food Consumption Among US Adults from 2001 to 2018." *American Journal of Clinical Nutrition* 115, no. 1 (January 2022): 211–21. https://doi.org/10.1093/ajcn/nqab305.

Kershaw, E., and J. Flier. "Adipose Tissue as an Endocrine Organ." *Journal of Clinical Endocrinology & Metabolism* 89, no. 6 (June 1, 2004): 2548–56. https://doi.org/10.1210/jc.2004-0395.

Komiya, S., Y. Naito, H. Okada, Y. Matsuo, K. Hirota, T. Takagi, K. Mizushima, R. Inoue, A. Abe, and Y. Morimoto. "Characterizing the Gut Microbiota in Females with Infertility and Preliminary Results of a Water-Soluble Dietary Fiber Intervention Study." *Journal of Clinical Biochemistry and Nutrition* 67, no. 1 (July 2020): 105–11. https://doi.org/10.3164/jcbn.20-53.

Kort, D. H., and R. A. Lobo. "Preliminary Evidence That Cinnamon Improves Menstrual Cyclicity in Women with Polycystic Ovary Syndrome: A Randomized Controlled Trial." *American Journal of Obstetrics and Gynecology* 211, no. 5 (November 1, 2014): 487. https://doi.org/10.1016/j.ajog.2014.05.009.

Lefèvre, P. L. C., M.F. Palin, and B. D. Murphy. "Polyamines on the Reproductive Landscape." *Endocrine Reviews* 32, no. 5 (October 1, 2011): 694–12. https://doi.org/10.1210/er.2011-0012.

Liu, Q., J. W. Y. Mak, Q. Su, Y. K. Yeoh, G. Chung-Yan Lui, S. So Shan Ng, F. Zhang, A. Y. L. Li, W. Lu, D. Shu-Cheong Hui, et al. "Gut Microbiota Dynamics in a Prospective Cohort of Patients with Post-Acute COVID-19 Syndrome." *BMJ Gut* 71, no. 3 (March 2022): 544–52. http://dx.doi.org/10.1136/gutjnl-2021-325989.

Lu, C., K. Toepel, R. Irish, R. A. Fenske, D. B. Barr, and R. Bravo. "Organic Diets Significantly Lower Children's Dietary Exposure to Organophosphorus Pesticides." *Environmental Health Perspectives* 114, no. 2 (February 1, 2006): 260–63. https://doi.org/10.1289/ehp.8418.

Ludwig, D. S., and C. B. Ebbeling. "The Carbohydrate-Insulin Model of Obesity: Beyond 'Calories In, Calories Out.'" *JAMA Internal*

Medicine 178, no. 8 (August 2018): 1098–103. https://doi.org/10.1001/jamainternmed.2018.2933.

Lyngsø, J., C. H. Ramlau-Hansen, B. Bay, H. J. Ingerslev, A. Hulman, and U. S. Kesmodel. "Association Between Coffee or Caffeine Consumption and Fecundity and Fertility: A Systematic Review and Dose-Response Meta-Analysis," *Clinical Epidemiology* 9, (December 15, 2017): 699–719. December 15, 2017, https://doi.org/10.2147/CLEP.S146496.

Maunder, A., E. Bessell, R. Lauche, J. Adams, A. Sainsbury, and N. Fuller. "Effectiveness of Herbal Medicines for Weight Loss: A Systematic Review and Meta-Analysis of Randomized Controlled Trials." *Diabetes, Obesity and Metabolism* 22, no. 6 (June 2020): 891–03. https://doi.org/10.1111/dom.13973.

McMillan, A. G., L. E. May, G. G. Gaines, C. Isler, and D. Kuehn. "Effects of Aerobic Exercise during Pregnancy on 1-Month Infant Neuromotor Skills." *Medicine & Science in Sports & Exercise* 51, no. 8 (August 2019): 1671–76. https://doi.org/10.1249/MSS.0000000000001958.

Munglue, P., S. Kupittayanant, and P. Kupittayanant. "Effect of Watermelon (Citrullus lanatus) Flesh Extract on Sexual Behavior of Male Rats." *Chiang Mai University Journal of Natural Sciences* 13, no. 1 (January 2014). https://doi.org/10.12982/CMUJNS.2014.0054.

Nettleton, J. A., P. L. Lutsey, Y. Wang, J. A. Lima, E. D. Michos, and D. R. Jacobs. "Diet Soda Intake and Risk of Incident Metabolic Syndrome and Type 2 Diabetes in the Multi-Ethnic Study of Atherosclerosis (MESA)." *Diabetes Care* 32, no. 4 (April 2009): 688–94. https://doi.org/10.2337/dc08-1799.

Norr, M., J. Hect, C. Lenniger, M. Van den Heuvel, and M. Thomason. "An Examination of Maternal Prenatal BMI and Human Fetal Brain Development." *Journal of Child Psychology and Psychiatry* 62, no. 4 (April 2021): 458–69. https://doi.org/10.1111/jcpp.13301.

Palmer, N., H. W. Bakos, T. Fullston, and M. Lane. "Impact of Obesity on Male Fertility, Sperm Function and Molecular Composition." *Spermatogenesis* 2, no. 4 (December 1, 2012): 253–63. https://doi.org/10.4161/spmg.21362.

Pilz, S., A. Zittermann, R. Obeid, A. Hahn, P. Pludowski, C. Trummer, E. Lerchbaum, F. R. Pérez-López, S. N. Karras, and W. März. "The Role of Vitamin D in Fertility and during Pregnancy and Lactation: A Review of Clinical Data." *International Journal of Environmental Research and Public Health* 15, no. 10 (October 12, 2018): 2241. https://doi.org/10.3390/ijerph15102241.

Qin, Y., A. S. Havulinna, Y. Liu, P. Jousilahti, S. C. Ritchie, A. Tokolyi,

J. G. Sanders, L. Valsta, M. Brożyńska, Q. Zhu, et al. "Combined Effects of Host Genetics and Diet on Human Gut Microbiota and Incident Disease in a Single Population Cohort." *Nature Genetics* 54, no. 2 (February 3, 2022): 134–42. https://doi.org/10.1038/s41588-021-00991-z.

Rahimipour, M., A. R. Talebi, M. Anvari, A. A. Sarcheshmeh, and M. Omidi. "Saccharin Consumption Increases Sperm DNA Fragmentation and Apoptosis in Mice." *Iranian Journal of Reproductive Medicine* 12, no. 5 (May 2014): 307–12.

Rahman, M., and A. Berenson. "Accuracy of Current Body Mass Index Obesity Classification for White, Black, and Hispanic Reproductive-Age Women." *Obstetrics & Gynecology* 115, no. 5 (May 2010): 982–88. https://doi.org/10.1097/AOG.0b013e3181da9423.

Ramlau-Hansen, C. H., A. M. Thulstrup, E. A. Nohr, J. P. Bonde, T. I. A. Sørensen, and J. Olsen. "Subfecundity in Overweight and Obese Couples." *Human Reproduction* 22, no. 6 (June 2007): 1634–37. https://doi.org/10.1093/humrep/dem035.

Ricci, E., S. Al-Beitawi, S. Cipriani, A. Alteri, F. Chiaffarino, M. Candiani, S. Gerli, P. Viganó, and F. Parazzini. "Dietary Habits and Semen Parameters: A Systematic Narrative Review." *Andrology* 6, no. 1 (January 2018): 104–16. https://doi.org/10.1111/andr.12452.

Traversy, G., and J-P. Chaput, "Alcohol Consumption and Obesity: An Update," *Current Obesity Reports* 4, no. 1 (December 2015): 122–30. https://link.springer.com/article/10.1007/s13679-014-0129-4.

Salas-Huetos, A., M. Bulló, and J. Salas-Salvadó. "Dietary Patterns, Foods and Nutrients in Male Fertility Parameters and Fecundability: A Systematic Review of Observational Studies." *Human Reproduction Update* 23, no. 4 (July–August 2017): 371–89. https://doi.org/10.1093/humupd/dmx006.

Skoracka, K., A. E. Ratajczak, A. M. Rychter, A. Dobrowolska, and I. Krela-Kaźmierczak. "Female Fertility and the Nutritional Approach: The Most Essential Aspects." *Advances in Nutrition* 12, no. 6 (November 2021): 2372–86. https://doi.org/10.1093/advances/nmab068.

Tasali, E., K. Wroblewski, E. Kahn, J. Kilkus, D. A. Schoeller. "Effect of Sleep Extension on Objectively Assessed Energy Intake among Adults with Overweight in Real-Life Settings: A Randomized Clinical Trial." *JAMA Internal Medicine* 182, no. 4 (February 7, 2022): 365–74. https://doi.org/10.1001/jamainternmed.2021.8098.

US Food and Drug Administration. "Guidance for Industry: Guide for Developing and Using Data Bases for Nutritional Labeling." FDA.

March 1998, updated September 20, 2018. https://www.fda.gov/regu latory-information/search-fda-guidance-documents/guidance-industry -guide-developing-and-using-data-bases-nutrition-labeling.

VandeVoort, C. A., K. N. Grimsrud, U. Midic, N. Mtango, and K. E. Latham. "Transgenerational Effects of Binge Drinking in a Primate Model: Implications for Human Health." *Fertility and Sterility*, 103, no. 2 (February 2015): 560–69. https://doi.org/10.1016/j .fertnstert.2014.10.051.

Van Heertum, K., and B. Rossi. "Alcohol and Fertility: How Much Is Too Much?" *Fertility Research and Practice* 3, no. 10 (July 10, 2017). https:// doi.org/10.1186/s40738-017-0037-x.

Vujkovic, M., J. Vries, J. Lindemans, P. van der Spek, E. Steegers, and R. Steegers-Theunissen. "The Preconception Mediterranean Dietary Pattern in Couples Undergoing In Vitro Fertilization/Intracytoplasmic Sperm Injection Treatment Increases the Chance of Pregnancy." *Fertility and Sterility* 94, no. 6 (November 1, 2010): 2096–101. https:// doi.org/10.1016/j.fertnstert.2009.12.079.

Wang, Y., C. Lehane, K. Ghebremeskel, and M. A. Crawford. "Modern Organic and Broiler Chickens Sold for Human Consumption Provide More Energy from Fat than Protein." *Public Health Nutrition* 13, no. 3 (March 2010): 400–08. https://doi.org/10.1017/S1368980009991157.

Wartella, E. A., A. H. Lichtenstein, and C. S. Boon, ed. "Chapter 2: History of Nutrition Labeling." In *Front-of-Package Nutrition Rating Systems and Symbols: Phase I Report*. Washington, DC: National Academies Press, 2010. https://www.ncbi.nlm.nih.gov/books/NBK209859.

Wasilewska, E., and S. Małgorzewicz. "Impact of Allergic Diseases on Fertility." *Advances in Dermatology and Allergology* 36, no. 5 (October 2019): 507–12. https://doi.org/10.5114/ada.2019.89501.

Wensink, M. J., Y. Lu, L. Tian, G. Shaw, S. Rizzi, T. K. Jensen, E. R. Mathiesen, N. E. Skakkebæk, R. Lindahl-Jacobsen, and M. L. Eisenberg. "Preconception Antidiabetic Drugs in Men and Birth Defects in Offspring: A Nationwide Cohort Study." *Annals of Internal Medicine* 175, no. 5 (May 2022): 665–73. https://doi.org/10.7326/M21-4389.

Wogatzky, J., B. Wirleitner, A. Stecher, P. Vanderzwalmen, A. Neyer, D. Spitzer, M. Schuff, B. Schechinger, and N. H. Zech. "The Combination Matters—Distinct Impact of Lifestyle Factors on Sperm Quality: A Study on Semen Analysis of 1683 Patients According to MSOME Criteria." *Reproductive Biology and Endocrinology* 10, no. 1 (December 2012): 115. https://doi .org/10.1186/1477-7827-10-115.

Zeevi, D., T. Korem, N. Zmora, D. Israeli, D. Rothschild, A. Weinberger, O. Ben-Yacov, D. Lador, T. Avnit-Sagi, M. Lotan-Pompan, et al. "Personalized Nutrition by Prediction of Glycemic Responses." *Cell* 163, no 5 (November 19, 2015): 1079–94. https://doi.org/10.1016/j.cell.2015.11.001.

CHAPTER 7: SUPPLEMENTS

"2017 CRN Consumer Survey on Dietary Supplements." CRN. Accessed September 13, 2022. https://www.crnusa.org/resources/2017-crn-consumer-survey-dietary-supplements.

Ahmadi, S., R. Bashiri, A. Ghadiri-Anari, and A. Nadjarzadeh. "Antioxidant Supplements and Semen Parameters: An Evidence Based Review." *International Journal of Reproductive Biomedicine* 14, no. 12 (December 2016): 729–36.

Bedaiwy, M. A., A. R. Al Inany, and T. Falcone. "N-acetyl Cystein Improves Pregnancy Rate in Long Standing Unexplained Infertility: A Novel Mechanism of Ovulation Induction." *Fertility and Sterility* 82, sup. 2 (September 1, 2004): S228. https://doi.org/10.1016/j.fertnstert.2004.07.604.

Boxmeer, J. C., M. Smit, E. Utomo, J. C. Romijn, M. J. C. Eijkemans, J. Lindemans, J. S. E. Laven, N. S. Macklon, E. A. P. Steegers, and R. P. M. Steegers-Theunissen. "Low Folate in Seminal Plasma Is Associated with Increased Sperm DNA Damage." *Fertility and Sterility* 92, no. 2, (August 1, 2009): 548–56. https://doi.org/10.1016/j.fertnstert.2008.06.010.

Chu, J., I. Gallos, A. Tobias, B. Tan, A. Eapen, and A. Coomarasamy. "Vitamin D and Assisted Reproductive Treatment Outcome: A Systematic Review and Meta-Analysis." *Human Reproduction* 33, no. 1 (January 2018): 65–80. https://doi.org/10.1093/humrep/dex326.

Crawford, T. J., C. A. Crowther, J. Alsweiler, and J. Brown. "Antenatal Dietary Supplementation with Myo-inositol in Women during Pregnancy for Preventing Gestational Diabetes." *Cochrane Database of Systematic Reviews*, no. 12 (December 2015): CD011507. https://doi.org/10.1002/14651858.CD011507.pub2.

de Ligny, W., R. M. Smits, R. Mackwnzie-Proctor, V. Jordan, K. Fleischer, J. P. de Bruin, and M. G. Showell. "Antioxidants for Male Subfertility." Cochrane Database of Systematic Reviews. May 4, 2022. https://doi.org/10.1002/14651858.CD007411.pub5.

"Dietary Supplements Market Size, Share & Trends Analysis Report by

Ingredient (Vitamins, Minerals), by Form, by Application, by End User, by Distribution Channel, by Region, and Segment Forecasts, 2022–2030." Grand View Research. Accessed September 13, 2022. https://www.grandviewresearch.com/industry-analysis/dietary-supplements-market.

Hall, K. T., J. Loscalzo, and T. J. Kaptchuk. "Genetics and the Placebo Effect: The Placebome." *Trends in Molecular Medicine* 21, no. 5 (May 1, 2015): 285–94. https://doi.org/10.1016/j.molmed.2015.02.009.

Jannatifar, R., K. Parivar, N. H. Roodbari, and M. H. Nasr-Esfahani. "Effects of N-Acetyl-Cysteine Supplementation on Sperm Quality, Chromatin Integrity and Level of Oxidative Stress in Infertile Men." *Reproductive Biology and Endocrinology* 17, no. 1 (February 2019): article 24. https://doi.org/10.1186/s12958-019-0468-9.

Jiang, Z., and H. Shen. "Mitochondria: Emerging Therapeutic Strategies for Oocyte Rescue." *Reproductive Sciences* 29, no. 3 (March 2022): 711–22. https://doi.org/10.1007/s43032-021-00523-4.

Klein, E. A., I. M. Thompson, C. M. Tangen, J. J. Crowley, M. S. Lucia, P. J. Goodman, L. M. Minasian, L. G. Ford, H. L. Parnes, J. M. Gaziano, et al. "Vitamin E and the Risk of Prostate Cancer: The Selenium and Vitamin E Cancer Prevention Trial (SELECT)." *JAMA* 306, no. 14 (October 12, 2011): 1549–56. https://doi.org/10.1001/jama.2011.1437.

Langsjoen, P. H., and A. M. Langsjoen. "Comparison Study of Plasma Coenzyme Q_{10} Levels in Healthy Subjects Supplemented with Ubiquinol versus Sbiquinone." *Clinical Pharmacology in Drug Development* 3, no. 1 (January 2014): 13–17. https://doi.org/10.1002/cpdd.73.

Merviel, P., P. James S. Bouée, M. Le Guillou, C. Rince, C. Nachtergaele, and V. Kerlan. "Impact of Myo-inositol Treatment in Women with Polycystic Ovary Syndrome in Assisted Reproductive Technologies." *Reproductive Health* 18, no. 13 (January 2021). https://doi.org/10.1186/s12978-021-01073-3.

Moslemi, M. K., and S. Tavanbakhsh. "Selenium–Vitamin E Supplementation in Infertile Men: Effects on Semen Parameters and Pregnancy Rate." *Internal Journal of General Medicine* 2011, no. 4 (January 23, 2011): 99–104. https://doi.org/10.2147/IJGM.S16275.

National Cancer Institute. "Selenium and Vitamin E Cancer Prevention Trial (SELECT): Questions and Answers." National Institutes of Health. Accessed September 13, 2022. https://www.cancer.gov/types/prostate/research/select-trial-results-qa.

Nenkova, G., L. Petrov, and A. Alexandrova. "Role of Trace Elements for

Oxidative Status and Quality of Human Sperm." *Balkan Medical Journal* 34, no. 4 (August 4, 2017): 343–48. https://doi.org/10.4274/balkanmedj.2016.0147.

Nouri, M., R. Amani, M. Nasr-Esfahani, and M. J. Tarrahi. "The Effects of Lycopene Supplement on the Spermatogram and Seminal Oxidative Stress in Infertile Men: A randomized, Double-Blind, Placebo-Controlled Clinical Trial." *Phytotherapy Research* 33, no. 12 (December 2019): 3203–11. https://doi.org/10.1002/ptr.6493.

Salve, J., S. Pate, K. Debnath, and D. Langade. "Adaptogenic and Anxiolytic Effects of Ashwagandha Root Extract in Healthy Adults: A Double-Blind, Randomized, Placebo-Controlled Clinical Study." *Cureus* 11, no. 12 (December 25, 2019): e6466. https://doi.org/10.7759/cureus.6466.

Tucker, J., T. Fischer, L. Upjohn, D. Mazzera, and M. Kumar. "Unapproved Pharmaceutical Ingredients Included in Dietary Supplements Associated with US Food and Drug Administration Warnings." *JAMA Network Open* 1, no. 6 (October 12, 2018): e183337, https://doi.org/10.1001/jamanetworkopen.2018.3337.

Wartolowska, K., A. Judge, S. Hopewell, G. S. Collins, B. J. F. Dean, I. Rombach, D. Brindley, J. Savulescu, D. J. Beard, and A. J. Carr. "Use of Placebo Controls in the Evaluation of Surgery: Systematic Review." *BMJ* 348 (May 2014): g3253. https://doi.org/10.1136/bmj.g3253.

Zhang, H., Z. Huang, L. Xiao, X. Jiang, D. Chen, and Y. Wei. "Meta-Analysis of the Effect of the Maternal Vitamin D Level on the Risk of Spontaneous Pregnancy Loss." *International Journal of Gynecology and Obstetrics* 138, no. 3 (September 2017): 242–49. https://doi.org/10.1002/ijgo.12209.

CHAPTER 8: EXERCISE

Chekroud, S. R., R. Gueorguieva, A. B. Zheutlin, M. Paulus, H. M. Krumholz, J. H. Krystal, and A. M. Chekroud. "Association between Physical Exercise and Mental Health in 1·2 Million Individuals in the USA between 2011 and 2015: A Cross-Sectional Study." *Lancet Psychiatry* 5, no. 9 (September 2018): 739–46. https://doi.org/10.1016/S2215-0366(18)30227-X.

Gaskins, A. J., J. Mendiola, M. Afeiche, N. Jørgensen, S. H. Swan, and J. E. Chavarro. "Physical Activity and Television Watching in Relation to Semen Quality in Young Men." *British Journal of Sports Medicine* 49, no. 4 (February 2015): 265–70. https://doi.org/10.1136/bjsports-2012-091644.

Gaskins, A. J., P. L. Williams, M. G. Keller, I. Souter, R. Hauser, and J. E. Chavarro. "Maternal Physical and Sedentary Activities in Relation to Reproductive Outcomes Following IVF." *Reproductive BioMedicine Online* 33, no. 4 (October 1, 2016): 513–21. https://doi.org/10.1016/j .rbmo.2016.07.002.

Hakimi, O., and L.C. Cameron. "Effect of Exercise on Ovulation: A Systematic Review." *Sports Medicine* 47, no. 8 (August 2017): 1555–67. https://doi.org/10.1007/s40279-016-0669-8.

Hurley, K. S., K. J. Flippin, L. C. Blom, J. E. Bolin, D. L. Hoover, and L. W. Judge. "Practices, Perceived Benefits, and Barriers to Resistance Training among Women Enrolled in College." *International Journal of Exercise Science* 11, no. 5 (May 2018): 226–38.

Jóźków, P., and M. Rossato. "The Impact of Intense Exercise on Semen Quality." *American Journal of Men's Health* 11, no. 3 (May 2017): 654–62. https://doi.org/10.1177/1557988316669045.

Keeler, J., M. Albrecht, L. Eberhardt, L. Horn, C. Donnelly, and D. Lowe. "Diastasis Recti Abdominis: A Survey of Women's Health Specialists for Current Physical Therapy Clinical Practice for Postpartum Women." *Journal of Women's Health Physical Therapy* 36, no. 3 (September/December 2012): 131–42. http://doi.org/10.1097 /JWH.0b013e318276f35f.

Laker, R. C., A. Altıntaş, T. S. Lillard, M. Zhang, J. J. Connelly, O. L. Sabik, S. Onengut, S. S. Rich, C. R. Farber, R. Barrès, Z. Yan. "Exercise during Pregnancy Mitigates Negative Efects of Parental Obesity on Metabolic Function in Adult Mouse Offspring." *Journal of Applied Physiology* 130, no. 3 (March 1, 2021): 605–16. https://doi.org/10.1152 /japplphysiol.00641.2020.

Maleki, H., and B. Tartibian. "Long-Term Low-to-Intensive Cycling Training: Impact on Semen Parameters and Seminal Cytokines." *Clinical Journal of Sport Medicine* 25, no. 6 (November 2015): 535–40. http:// doi.org/10.1097/JSM.0000000000000122.

Sato, S., K. A. Dyar, J. T. Treebak, S. L. Jepsen, A. M. Ehrlich, S. P. Ashcroft, K. Trost, T. Kunzke, V. M. Prade, L. Small, et al. "Atlas of Exercise Metabolism Reveals Time-Dependent Signatures of Metabolic Homeostasis." *Cell Metabolism* 34, no. 2 (February 1, 2022): 329–45. e8. https://doi.org/10.1016/j.cmet.2021.12.016.

Thom, D. H., and G. Rortveit. "Prevalence of Postpartum Urinary Incontinence: A Systematic Review." *Acta Obstetricia et Gynecologica Scandinavica* 89, no. 12 (December 2010): 1511–22. https://doi.org/10 .3109/00016349.2010.526188.

Wahl, K.J., N. L. Orr, M. Lisonek, H. Noga, M. A. Bedaiwy, C. Williams, C. Allaire, A. Y. Albert, K. B. Smith, S. Cox, and P. J. Yong. "Deep Dyspareunia, Superficial Dyspareunia, and Infertility Concerns among Women with Endometriosis: A Cross-Sectional Study." *Sexual Medicine* 8, no. 2 (June 1, 2020): 274–81. https://doi.org/10.1016/j .esxm.2020.01.002.

Williams, N. "The Borg Rating of Perceived Exertion (RPE) Scale." *Occupational Medicine* 67, no. 5 (July 2017): 404–05. https://doi .org/10.1093/occmed/kqx063.

Woodward, A., M. Klonizakis, and D. Broom. "Exercise and Polycystic Ovary Syndrome." *Physical Exercise for Human Health. Advances in Experimental Medicine and Biology* 1228 (2020): 123–36. https://doi .org/10.1007/978-981-15-1792-1_8.

Zhuo, Z., C. Wang, H. Yu, and J. Li. "The Relationship Between Pelvic Floor Function and Sexual Function in Perimenopausal Women." *Sexual Medicine* 9, no. 6 (December 1, 2021): 100441. https://doi .org/10.1016/j.esxm.2021.100441.

CHAPTER 9: CHEMICALS, DRUGS, AND THE ENVIRONMENT

Almond, D., and J. Currie. "Killing Me Softly: The Fetal Origins Hypothesis." *Journal of Economic Perspectives* 25, no. 3 (Summer 2011): 153–72. https://doi.org/10.1257/jep.25.3.153.

Alwan, S., and C. D. Chambers. "Identifying Human Teratogens: An Update." *Journal of Pediatric Genetics* 4, no. 2 (June 2015): 39–41. https://doi .org/10.1055/s-0035-1556745.

Auger, N., W. D. Fraser, R. Sauve, M. Bilodeau-Bertrand, and T. Kosatsky. "Risk of Congenital Heart Defects after Ambient Heat Exposure Early in Pregnancy." *Environmental Health Perspectives* 125, no. 1 (January 2017): 8–14. https://doi.org/10.1289/EHP171.

Baranger, D. A. A., S. E. Paul, S. M. C. Colbert, N. R. Karcher, E. C. Johnson, A. S. Hatoum, and R. Bogdan. "Association of Mental Health Burden with Prenatal Cannabis Exposure from Childhood to Early Adolescence: Longitudinal Findings from the Adolescent Brain Cognitive Development (ABCD) Study." *JAMA Pediatrics.* September 12, 2022. http://doi.org/10.1001/jamapediatrics.2022.3191.

Brin, M. F., R. S. Kirby, A. Slavotinek, M. A. Miller-Messana, L. Parker, I. Yushmanova, and H. Yang. "Pregnancy Outcomes Following Exposure to OnabotulinumtoxinA." *Pharmacoepidemiology and Drug*

Safety 25, no. 2 (December 2015): 179–87. https://doi.org/10.1002/pds.3920.

Buckley, J. P., J. R. Kuiper, D. H. Bennett, E. S. Barrett, T. Bastain, C. V. Breton, S. Chinthakindi, A. L. Dunlop, S. F. Farzan, J. B. Herbstman, et al. "Exposure to Contemporary and Emerging Chemicals in Commerce among Pregnant Women in the United States: The Environmental Influences on Child Health Outcome (ECHO) Program." *Environmental Science & Technology* 56, no. 10 (2022): 6560–73. http://doi.org/10.1021/acs.est.1c08942.

Carré, J., N. Gatimel, J. Moreau, J. Parinaud, and R. Léandri. "Does Air Pollution Play a Role in Infertility? A Systematic Review." *Environmental Health* 16, no. 1 (July 2017): article 82. https://doi.org/10.1186/s12940-017-0291-8.

Edelman, A., E. Boniface, E. Benhar, L. Han, K. A. Matteson, C. Favaro, J. Pearson, and B. Darney. "Association between Menstrual Cycle Length and Coronavirus Disease 2019 (COVID-19) Vaccination: A U.S. Cohort." *Obstetrics & Gynecology* 139, no. 4 (April 2022): 481–89. http://doi.org/10.1097/AOG.0000000000004695.

Edwards, L., N. L. McCray, B. N. VanNoy, A. Yau, R. J. Geller, G. Adamkiewicz, and A. R. Zota. "Phthalate and Novel Plasticizer Concentrations in Food Items from U.S. Fast Food Chains: A Preliminary Analysis." *Journal of Exposure Science & Environmental Epidemiology* 32 (May 2022): 366–73. https://doi.org/10.1038/s41370-021-00392-8.

Gaál, A., and G. Csaba. "Testosterone and Progesterone Level Alterations in the Adult Rat after Retinoid (Retinol or Retinoic Acid) Treatment (Imprinting) in Neonatal or Adolescent Age." *Hormone and Metabolic Research* 30, no. 8 (August 1998): 487–89. https://doi.org/10.1055/s-2007-978917.

Hallegraeff, G. M., D. M. Anderson, C. Belin, M.Y. Dechraoui Bottein, E. Bresnan, M. Chinain, H. Enevoldsen, M. Iwataki, B. Karlson, C. H. McKenzie, et al. "Perceived Global Increase in Algal Blooms Is Attributable to Intensified Monitoring and Emerging Bloom Impacts." *Communications Earth & Environment* 2, no. 1 (June 2021): 117. https://doi.org/10.1038/s43247-021-00178-8.

Harley, K. G., K. Kogut, D. S. Madrigal, M. Cardenas, I. A. Vera, G. Meza-Alfaro, J. She, Q. Gavin, R. Zahedi, A. Bradman, et al. "Reducing Phthalate, Paraben, and Phenol Exposure from Personal Care Products in Adolescent Girls: Findings from the HERMOSA Intervention Study." *Environmental Health Perspectives* 124, no. 10 (October 2016): 1600–07. https://doi.org/10.1289/ehp.1510514.

Huo, X., D. Chen, Y. He, W. Zhu, W. Zhou, and J. Zhang. "Bisphenol-A and Female Infertility: A Possible Role of Gene-Environment Interactions." *International Journal of Environmental Research and Public Health* 12, no. 9 (September 2015): 11101-116. https://doi.org/10.3390/ijerph120911101.

Jahnke, S. A., W. Poston, N. Jitnarin, C. K. Haddock. "Maternal and Child Health Among Female Firefighters in the US." *Maternal and Child Health Journal* 22, no. 6, (June 2018): 922–931. https://doi.org/10.1007/s10995-018-2468-3.

Jayasena, C. N., U. K. Radia, M. Figueiredo, L. F. Revill, A. Dimakopoulou, M. Osagie, W. Vessey, L. Regan, R. Raj, W. S. Dhillo. "Reduced Testicular Steroidogenesis and Increased Semen Oxidative Stress in Male Partners as Novel Markers of Recurrent Miscarriage." *Clinical Chemistry* 65, no. 1 (January 1, 2019): 161–69. https://doi.org/10.1373/clinchem.2018.289348.

Koman, P. D., K. A. Hogan, N. Sampson, R. Mandell, C. M. Coombe, M. M. Tetteh, Y. R. Hill-Ashford, D. Wilkins, M. G. Zlatnik, R. Loch-Caruson, et al. "Examining Joint Effects of Air Pollution Exposure and Social Determinants of Health in Defining 'At-Risk' Populations Under the Clean Air Act: Susceptibility of Pregnant Women to Hypertensive Disorders of Pregnancy." *World Medical & Health Policy* 10, no. 1 (March 2018): 7–54. https://doi.org/10.1002/wmh3.257.

Leslie, H. A., M. J. M. van Velzen, S. H. Brandsma, A. D. Vethaak, J. J. Garcia-Vallejo, M. H. Lamoree. "Discovery and Quantification of Plastic Particle Pollution in Human Blood." *Environment International* 163 (May 2022): 107199. https://doi.org/10.1016/j.envint.2022.107199.

Liu, J., and J. W. Martin. "Prolonged Exposure to Bisphenol A from Single Dermal Contact Events." *Environmental Science & Technology* 51, no. 17 (September 2017): 9940–49. https://doi.org/10.1021/acs.est.7b03093.

Luoma, Jon. "Challenged Conceptions: Environmental Chemicals and Fertility." October 2005. https://www.healthandenvironment.org/uploads-old/Challenged_Conceptions.pdf.

Mnif, W., A. I. H. Hassine, A. Bouaziz, A. Bartegi, O. Thomas, and B. Roig. "Effect of Endocrine Disruptor Pesticides: A Review." *International Journal of Environmental Research and Public Health* 8, no. 6 (June 2011): 2265–303. https://doi.org/10.3390/ijerph8062265.

Nowak, K., W. Ratajczak-Wrona, M. Górska, and E. Jabłońska. "Parabens and Their Effects on the Endocrine System." *Molecular and*

Cellular Endocrinology 474 (October 15, 2018): 238–51. https://doi
.org/10.1016/j.mce.2018.03.014.

Petersen, K. U., J. Hansen, N. E. Ebbehoej, J. P. Bonde. "Infertility in a
Cohort of Male Danish Firefighters: A Register-Based Study." *American
Journal of Epidemiology* 188, no. 2 (February 2019): 339–46. https://
doi.org/10.1093/aje/kwy235.

Pizzorno, J. "Environmental Toxins and Infertility." *Integrative Medicine* 17,
no. 2 (April 2018): 8–11.

Pomeroy, Reina. "Climate Change and Fertility: A Modern Survey of 2800+
People with Ovaries." *A Modern Fertility Blog.* December 1, 2021.
https://modernfertility.com/blog/climate-change-and-fertility-survey/.

Qiu, L., M. Chen, X. Wang, S. Chen, and Z. Ying. "$PM_{2.5}$ Exposure of
Mice during Spermatogenesis: A Role of Inhibitor κB Kinase 2 in Pro-
Opiomelanocortin Neurons." *Environmental Health Perspectives* 129,
no. 9 (September 2021). https://doi.org/10.1289/EHP8868.

Ragusa, A., A. Svelato, C. Santacroce, P; Catalano, V. Notarstefano, O.
Carnevali, F. Papa, M. C. A. Rongioletti, F. Baiocco, S. Draghi, et
al. "Plasticenta: First Evidence of Microplastics in Human Placenta."
Environment International 146 (January 2021): 106274. https://doi
.org/10.1016/j.envint.2020.106274.

Rahman, MD, S., W.-S. Kwon, J.-S. Lee, S.-J. Yoon, B.-Y. Ryu, and M.-G.
Pang. "Bisphenol-A Affects Male Fertility via Fertility-Related Proteins
in Spermatozoa." *Scientific Reports* 5 (2015): 9169. https://doi.org
/10.1038/srep09169.

Rotondo, E., and F. Chiarelli. "Endocrine-Disrupting Chemicals and Insulin
Resistance in Children." *Biomedicines* 8, no. 6 (May 2020): 137.
https://doi.org/10.3390/biomedicines8060137.

Rundle, A., L. Hoepner, A. Hassoun, S. Oberfield, G. Freyer, D. Holmes, M. Reyes,
J. Quinn, D. Camann, F. Perera, et al. "Association of Childhood Obesity
with Maternal Exposure to Ambient Air Polycyclic Aromatic Hydrocarbons
during Pregnancy." *American Journal of Epidemiology* Volume 175, no. 11
(June 2012): 1163–72. https://doi.org/10.1093/aje/kwr455.

Wesselink, A. K., E. E. Hatch, K. J. Rothman, T. R. Wang, M. D. Willis, J.
Yland, H. M. Crowe, R. J. Geller, S. K. Willis, R. B. Perkins, et al.
"A Prospective Cohort Study of COVID-19 Vaccination, SARS-CoV-2
Infection, and Fertility." *American Journal of Epidemiology* 191, no. 8
(August 2022): 1383–95. https://doi.org/10.1093/aje/kwac011.

"What You Should Know about When Using Cannabis, Including CBD,
When Pregnant or Breastfeeding." US Food and Drug Administration.
Accessed September 12, 2022. https://www.fda.gov/consumers/con

sumer-updates/what-you-should-know-about-using-cannabis-includ
ing-cbd-when-pregnant-or-breastfeeding.

Zhang, L., L. Dong, S. Ding, P. Qiao, C. Wang, M. Zhang, L. Zhang,
Q. Du, Y. Li, N. Tang, and B. Chang. "Effects of n-butylparaben
on Steroidogenesis and Spermatogenesis through Changed E_2
Levels in Male Rat Offspring." *Environmental Toxicology and
Pharmacology* 37, no. 2 (May 2014): 705–17. https://doi.org/10.1016/j
.etap.2014.01.016.

CHAPTER 10: MENTAL HEALTH

American Psychological Association. "Stress in America™ 2020: A National
Mental Health Crisis." Accessed September 12, 2022. https://www.apa
.org/news/press/releases/stress/2020/report-october.

Asmussen, S., D. M. Maybauer, J. D. Chen, J. D. Fraser, M. H. Toon,
R. Przkora, K. Jennings, M. O. Maybauer. "Effects of Acupuncture in
Anesthesia for Craniotomy: A Meta-Analysis." *Journal of Neurosurgical
Anesthesiology* 29, no. 3 (July 2017): 219–27. https://doi.org/10.1097
/ANA.0000000000000290.

Beeder, L. A., and M. K. Samplaski. "Effect of Antidepressant Medications
on Semen Parameters and Male Fertility." *International Journal of
Urology* 27, no. 1 (September 21, 2019): 39–46. https://doi.org/10.1111
/iju.14111.

Berretz, G., C. Cebula, B. M. Wortelmann, P. Papadopoulou, O. T. Wolf,
S. Ocklenburg, J. Packheiser. "Romantic Partner Embraces Reduce
Cortisol Release after Acute Stress Induction in Women but Not
in Men." *PLoS ONE* 17, no. 5 (May 2022): e0266887. https://doi
.org/10.1371/journal.pone.0266887.

Boccia, M., L. Piccardi, and P. Guariglia. "The Meditative Mind: A
Comprehensive Meta-Analysis of MRI Studies." *BioMed Research
International* 2015 (June 2015): article 419808. https://doi
.org/10.1155/2015/419808.

Charlet, K., and A. Heinz. "Harm Reduction—A Systematic Review on
Effects of Alcohol Reduction on Physical and Mental Symptoms."
Addiction Biology 22, no. 5 (June 2016): 1119–59. https://doi
.org/10.1111/adb.12414.

Choy, J. T., and M. L. Eisenberg. "Comprehensive Men's Health and Male
Infertility." *Translational Andrology and Urology* 9, supp. 2 (March
2020): S239–43. https://doi.org/10.21037/tau.2019.08.35.

Domar, A. D., V. A. Moragianni, D. A. Ryley, and A. C. Urato. "The Risks of Selective Serotonin Reuptake Inhibitor Use in Infertile Women: A Review of the Impact on Fertility, Pregnancy, Neonatal Health and Beyond." *Human Reproduction* 28, no. 1 (January 2013): 160–71. https://doi.org/10.1093/humrep/des383.

Ford, E. S., T. J. Cunningham, and J. B. Croft. "Trends in Self-Reported Sleep Duration among US Adults from 1985 to 2012." *Sleep* 38, no. 5 (May 1, 2015): 829–32. https://doi.org/10.5665/sleep.4684.

Frick, L. R., M. L. Arcos, M. Rapanelli, M. P. Zappia, M. Brocco, C. Mongini, A. M. Genaro, and G. A. Cremaschi. "Chronic Restraint Stress Impairs T-cell Immunity and Promotes Tumor Progression in Mice." *Stress* 12, no. 2 (March 2009): 134–43. https://doi.org/10.1080/10253890802137437.

Guyot, E., J. Baudry, S. Hercberg, P. Galan, E. Kesse-Guyot, and S. Péneau. "Mindfulness Is Associated with the Metabolic Syndrome among Individuals with a Depressive Symptomatology." *Nutrients* 10, no. 2 (February 2018): 232. https://doi.org/10.3390/nu10020232.

Hofmeister, S., and S. Bodden. "Premenstrual Syndrome and Premenstrual Dysphoric Disorder." *American Family Physician* 94, no. 3 (August 1, 2016): 236–40.

Kiecolt-Glaser, J. K., D. L. Habash, C. P. Fagundes, R. Andridge, J. Peng, W. B. Malarkey, M. A. Belury. "Daily Stressors, Past Depression, and Metabolic Responses to High-Fat Meals: A Novel Path to Obesity." *Biological Psychiatry* 77, no. 7 (April 1, 2015): 653–60. https://doi.org/10.1016/j.biopsych.2014.05.018.

Luppino, F. S., L. M. de Wit, P. F. Bouvy, T. Stijnen, P. Cuijpers, B. W. Penninx, and F. G. Zitman. "Overweight, Obesity, and Depression: A Systematic Review and Meta-Analysis of Longitudinal Studies." *Archives of General Psychiatry* 67, no. 3 (March 2010): 220–229. https://doi.org/10.1001/archgenpsychiatry.2010.2.

Lynch, C. D., R. Sundaram, J. M. Maisog, A. M. Sweeney, and G. M. Buck Louis."Preconception Stress Increases the Risk of Infertility: Results from a Couple-Based Prospective Cohort Study—The LIFE Study." *Human Reproduction* 29, no. 5 (May 2014): 1067–75. https://doi.org/10.1093/humrep/deu032.

Ma, S. H., and J. D. Teasdale. "Mindfulness-Based Cognitive Therapy for Depression: Replication and Exploration of Differential Relapse Prevention Effects." *Journal of Consulting and Clinical Psychology* 72, no. 1 (February 2004): 31–40. https://doi.org/10.1037/0022-006X.72.1.31.

Mikkelsen, K., L. Stojanovska, M. Polenakovic, M. Bosevski, and V.

Apostolopoulos. "Exercise and Mental Health." *Maturitas* 106 (December 2017): 48–56. https://doi.org/10.1016/j.maturitas.2017.09.003.

Oh, H., A. Koyanagi, J. E. DeVylder, and A. Stickley. "Seasonal Allergies and Psychiatric Disorders in the United States." *International Journal of Environmental Research and Public Health* 15, no. 9 (2018): 1965. https://doi.org/10.3390/ijerph15091965.

Peterson, B., J. Boivin, J. Norré, C. Smith, P. Thorn, and T. Wischmann. "An Introduction to Infertility Counseling: A Guide for Mental Health and Medical Professionals." *Journal of Assisted Reproduction and Genetics* 29, no. 3 (March 2012): 243–48. https://doi.org/10.1007 /s10815-011-9701-y.

Sansone, R. A., and L. A. Sansone. "Sunshine, Serotonin, and Skin: A Partial Explanation for Seasonal Patterns in Psychopathology?" *Innovations in Clinical Neuroscience* 10, no. 7 (July–August 2013): 20–24.

Sheng, J. A., N. J. Bales, S. A. Myers, A. I. Bautista, M. Roueinfar, T. M. Hale, R. J. Handa. "The Hypothalamic-Pituitary-Adrenal Axis: Development, Programming Actions of Hormones, and Maternal-Fetal Interactions." *Frontiers in Behavioral Neuroscience* 13 (January 2021). https://doi .org/10.3389/fnbeh.2020.601939.

Shobeiri, F., F. E. Araste, R. Ebrahimi, E. Jenabi, and M. Nazari. "Effect of Calcium on Premenstrual Syndrome: A Double-Blind Randomized Clinical Trial." *Obstetrics & Gynecology Science* 60, no. 1 (January 2017): 100–05. https://doi.org/10.5468/ogs.2017.60.1.100.

Song, C., H. Ikei, T. Kagawa, and Y. Miyazaki. "Effects of Walking in a Forest on Young Women." *International Journal of Environmental Research and Public Health* 16, no. 2 (January 2019): 229. https://doi .org/10.3390/ijerph16020229.

Tzeng, N.-S., H.-A. Chang, C.-H. Chung, Y.-C. Kao, C.-C. Chang, H.-W. Yeh, W.-S. Chiang, Y.-C. Chou, S.-Y. Chang, W.-C Chien. "Increased Risk of Psychiatric Disorders in Allergic Diseases: A Nationwide, Population-Based, Cohort Study." *Frontiers in Psychiatry* 9 (April 2018): article 133. https://doi.org/10.3389/fpsyt.2018.00133.

Xie, Y., Q. Tang, G. Chen, M. Xie, S. Yu, J. Zhao, and L. Chen. "New Insights into the Circadian Rhythm and Its Related Diseases." *Frontiers in Physiology* 10, June 25, 2019: 682. https://doi.org/10.3389/fphys.2019.0068.

CHAPTER 11: MAKING BABIES

Aron, A., E. N. Aron, and D. Smollan. "Inclusion of Other in the Self Scale and the Structure of Interpersonal Closeness." *Journal of Personality and Social Psychology* 63, no. 4 (1992): 596–612. https://doi.org /10.1037/0022-3514.63.4.596.

Coonrod, D. V., B. W. Jack, K. A. Boggess, R. Long, J. A. Conry, S. N. Cox, R. Cefalo, K. D. Hunter, A. Pizzica, and A. L. Dunlop. "The Clinical Content of Preconception Care: Immunizations as Part of Preconception Care," *AJOG* 199, no. 6, supp. B (December 1, 2008): S290-S295. https://doi.org/10.1016/j.ajog.2008.08.061.

Herbenick, D., M. Rosenberg, L. Golzarri-Arroyo, J. D. Fortenberry, and T.-C. Fu. "Changes in Penile-Vaginal Intercourse Frequency and Sexual Repertoire from 2009 to 2018: Findings from the National Survey of Sexual Health and Behavior." *Archives of Sexual Behavior* 51, no. 3 (November 2021): 1419–33. https://doi.org/10.1007/s10508-021-02125-2.

Lamb, Robert. "Scientists Once Dressed Frogs in Tiny Pants to Study Reproduction." *Atlas Obscura*. September 18, 2017. https://www.at lasobscura.com/articles/frog-pants-reproduction-experiment.

National Health Service. "How Long Does It Usually Take to Get Pregnant?" Accessed September 12, 2022. https://www.nhs.uk/pregnancy /trying-for-a-baby/how-long-it-takes-to-get-pregnant/.

"Pasteur and Spontaneous Generation." In *Microbiology* (online textbook). Boundless: January 3, 2021. https://bio.libretexts.org/Bookshelves /Microbiology/Book%3A_Microbiology_(Boundless)/1%3A _Introduction_to_Microbiology/1.1%3A_Introduction_to _Microbiology/1.1C%3A_Pasteur_and_Spontaneous_Generation.

CHAPTER 12: FERTILITY TESTING

Agarwal, A., A. Majzoub, S. C. Esteves, E. Ko, R. Ramasamy, and A. Zini. "Clinical Utility of Sperm DNA Fragmentation Testing: Practice Recommendations Based on Clinical Scenarios." *Translational Andrology and Urology* 5, no. 6 (December 2016): 935–50. https://doi .org/10.21037/tau.2016.10.03.

Bassil, R., R. Casper, N. Samara, T.-B. Hsieh, E. Barzilay, R. Orvieto, and J. Haas. "Does the Endometrial Receptivity Array Really Provide Personalized Embryo Transfer?" *Journal of Assisted Reproduction and Genetics* 35, no. 7 (July 2018): 1301–05. https://doi.org/10.1007 /s10815-018-1190-9.

Centers for Disease Control and Prevention. "[Assisted Reproductive Technology] ART Success Rates." US Department of Health and Human Services. Accessed September 12, 2022, https://www.cdc.gov /art/artdata/index.html.

Enabnit, Alex. "We Asked 500 People, 'Do You Lie to Your Doctor?'" TermLife2Go. February 24, 2020. https://termlife2go.com/lying-to-your-doctor/.

"Fertility Test Market Worth $680 Million by 2025." Markets and Markets. Accessed September 12, 2022. https://www.marketsandmarkets.com/PressReleases/fertility-testing-devices.asp.

Flemming, R. "The Invention of Infertility in the Classical Greek World: Medicine, Divinity, and Gender." *Bulletin of the History of Medicine* 87, no. 4 (Winter 2013): 565–90. https://doi.org/10.1353/bhm.2013.0064.

Garolla, A., D. Pizzol, and C. Foresta. "The Role of Human Papillomavirus on Sperm Function." *Current Opinion in Obstetrics and Gynecology* 23, no. 4 (August 2011): 232–237. https://doi.org/10.1097/GCO.0b013e328348a3a4.

Gnoth, C., D. Godehardt, E. Godehardt, P. Frank Herrmann, and G. Freundl. "Time to Pregnancy: Results of the German Prospective Study and Impact on the Management of Infertility." *Human Reproduction* 18, no. 9 (September 2003): 1959–66. https://doi.org/10.1093/humrep/deg366.

Hansen, K. A., and K. M. Eyster. "Genetics and Genomics of Endometriosis." *Clinical Obstetrics and Gynecology* 53, no. 2 (June 2010): 403–12. https://doi.org/10.1097/GRF.0b013e3181db7ca.

Kantartzi, P. D., C. D. Goulis, G. D. Goulis, and I. Papadimas. "Male Infertility and Varicocele: Myths and Reality." *Hippokratia* 11, no. 3 (July–September 2007): 99–104.

Khan, M. J., A. Ullah, and S. Basit. "Genetic Basis of Polycystic Ovary Syndrome (PCOS): Current Perspectives." *Application of Clinical Genetics* 12 (December 2019): 249–60. https://doi.org/10.2147/TACG.S200341.

Martin, E., J. B. Carnett, J. V. Levi, and M. E. Pennington. "The Surgical Treatment of Sterility Due to Obstruction at the Epididymis; Together with a Study of the Morphology of Human Spermatozoa." *University of Pennsylvania Medical Bulletin* 15, no. 1 (March 1902): 2–15.

Pereira, N., K. M. Kucharczyk, J. L. Estes, R. S. Gerber, J. P. Lekovich, R. T. Elias, and S. D. Spandorfer. "Human Papillomavirus Infection, Infertility, and Assisted Reproductive Outcomes." *Journal of Pathogens* 2015 (November 2015): 578423. https://doi.org/10.1155/2015/578423.

Quaas, A., and A. Dokras. "Diagnosis and Treatment of Unexplained Infertility." *Reviews in Obstetrics & Gynecology* 1, no. 2 (Spring 2008): 69–76.

Rahban, R., L. Priskorn, A. Senn, E. Stettler, F. Galli, J. Vargas, M. Van den Bergh, A. Fusconi, R. Garlantezec, T. K. Jensen, et al. "Semen Quality of Young Men in Switzerland: A Nationwide Cross-Sectional Population-Based Study." *Andrology* 7, no. 6 (November 2019): 818–26. https://doi.org/10.1111/andr.12645.

Riera-Escamilla, A., M. Vockel, L. Nagirnaja, M. J. Xavier, A. Carbonell, D. Moreno-Mendoza, M. Pybus, G. Farnetani, V. Rosta, F. Cioppi, et al. "Large-Scale Analyses of the X Chromosome in 2,354 Infertile Men Discover Recurrently Affected Genes Associated with Spermatogenic Failure," *Cell* 109, no. 8 (August 4, 2022): 1458–71. https://doi.org/10.1016/j.ajhg.2022.06.007.

Ruiz-Alonso, M., N. Galindo, A. Pellicer, and C. Simón. "What a Difference Two Days Make: 'Personalized' Embryo Transfer (pET) Paradigm: A Case Report and Pilot Study." *Human Reproduction* 29, no. 6 (June 2014): 1244–47. https://doi.org/10.1093/humrep/deu070.

Van Welie, N., K. Rosielle, K. Dreyer, J. Rijswijk, C. B. Lambalk, N. van Geloven, V. Mijatovic, B. W. J. Mol, and R. van Eekelen. "How Long Does the Fertility-Enhancing Effect of Hysterosalpingography with Oil-Based Contrast Last?" *Reproductive BioMedicine Online* 41, no. 6 (December 1, 2020): 1038–44. https://doi.org/10.1016/j.rbmo.2020.08.038.

World Health Organization. "WHO Laboratory Manual for the Examination and Processing of Human Semen." Sixth Edition. July 27, 2021. https://www.who.int/publications/i/item/9789240030787.

CHAPTER 13: FERTILITY PRESERVATION

Diaz, P., J. Zizzo, N. C. Balaji, R. Reddy, K. Khodamoradi, J. Ory, and R. Ramasamy. "Fear about Adverse Effect on Fertility Is a Major Cause of COVID-19 Vaccine Hesitancy in the United States." *Andrologia* 54, no. 4 (December 30, 2021): e14361. https://doi.org/10.1111/and.14361.

Elizalde, Molly, "How Egg Freezing Went Mainstream." *New York Times.* April 17, 2020. https://www.nytimes.com/2020/04/17/parenting/fertility/egg-freezing.html.

Fertility and Sterility Editorial Office. "Fertility Considerations: The COVID-19 Disease May Have a More Negative Impact than the COVID-19 Vaccine, Especially among Men." American Society for Reproductive Medicine. March 19, 2021. https://www.fertstertdialog.com/posts/fertility-considerations-the-covid-19-disease-may-have-a-more-negative-impact-than-the-covid-19-vaccine-especially-among-men?room_id=871-covid-19.

FertilityIQ. "Egg Freezing." https://www.fertilityiq.com/egg-freezing/the-costs
-of-egg-freezing.

Goldman, R. H., C. Racowsky, L. V. Farland, S. Munné, L. Ribustello, and
J. H. Fox. "Predicting the Likelihood of Live Birth for Elective Oocyte
Cryopreservation: A Counseling Tool for Physicians and Patients."
Human Reproduction 32, no. 4 (April 2017): 853–59. https://doi
.org/10.1093/humrep/dex008.

Huang, C., L. Lei, H.-L. Wu, R.-X. Gan, Z.-B. Yuan, L.Q. Fan, W.-B. Zhu.
"Long-Term Cryostorage of Semen in a Human Sperm Bank Does not
Affect Clinical Outcomes." *Fertility and Sterility* 112, no. 4 (October 1,
2019): 663–69. https://doi.org/10.1016/j.fertnstert.2019.06.008.

Inhorn, M. C., D. Birenbaum-Carmeli, L. M. Westphal, J. Doyle, N. Gleicher,
D. Meirow, M. Dirnfeld, D. Seidman, A. Kahane, P, Patrizio. "Ten
Pathways to Elective Egg Freezing: A Binational Analysis." *Journal
of Assisted Reproduction and Genetics* 32, no. 11 (November 2008):
2003–11. https://doi.org/10.1007/s10815-018-1277-3.

Lampert, Natalie. "The Unexpected Freedom That Comes with Freezing
Your Eggs." *New York Times*. December 11, 2019. https://www.ny
times.com/2019/12/11/magazine/egg-freezing-fertility.html.

Leung, A., D. Sakkas, S. Pang, K. Thornton, and N. Resetkova. "Assisted
Reproductive Technology Outcomes in Female-to-Male Transgender
Patients Compared with Cisgender Patients: A New Frontier in
Reproductive Medicine." *Fertility and Sterility* 112, no. 5 (November
1, 2019): 858–65. https://doi.org/10.1016/j.fertnstert.2019.07.014.

Pacheco, F., and K. Oktay. "Current Success and Efficiency of Autologous
Ovarian Transplantation: A Meta-Analysis." *Reproductive Sciences* 24,
no. 8 (August 2017): 1111–20. https://doi.org/10.1177/1933719117702.

Rienzi, L., C. Gracia, R. Maggiulli, A. R. LaBarbera, D. J. Kaser, F. M. Ubaldi,
S. Vanderpoel, and C. Racowsky. "Oocyte, Embryo and Blastocyst
Cryopreservation in ART: Systematic Review and Meta-Analysis
Comparing Slow-Freezing versus Vitrification to Produce Evidence
for the Development of Global Guidance." *Human Reproduction
Update* 23, no. 2 (March–April 2017): 139–55. https://doi.org/10.1093
/humupd/dmw038.

Valli-Pulaski, H., K. A. Peters, K. Gassei, S. R. Steimer, M. Sukhwani, B.
P. Hermann, L. Dwomor, S. David, A. P. Fayomi, S. K. Munyoki, et
al. "Testicular Tissue Cryopreservation: 8 Years of Experience from
a Coordinated Network of Academic Centers." *Human Reproduction*
34, no. 6 (June 2019): 966–77. https://doi.org/10.1093/humrep
/dez043.

CHAPTER 14: FERTILITY TREATMENT AND ASSISTED REPRODUCTION

Arocho, R., E. B. Lozano, and C. T. Halpern. "Estimates of Donated Sperm Use in the United States: National Survey of Family Growth 1995–2017." *Fertility and Sterility* 112, no. 4 (October 1, 2019): 718–23. https://doi.org/10.1016/j.fertstert.2019.05.031.

Bowles, Nellie. "The Sperm Kings Have a Problem: Too Much Demand." *New York Times*. January 8, 2021, updated January 20, 2021. https://www.nytimes.com/2021/01/08/business/sperm-donors-facebook-groups.html.

Carmichael, S. L., and G. M. Shaw. "Maternal Corticosteroid Use and Risk of Selected Congenital Anomalies." *American Journal of Medical Genetics* 86, no. 3 (September 1999): 242–44. https://pubmed.ncbi.nlm.nih.gov/10482873/.

Craciunas, L., N. Tsampras, N. Raine Fenning, and A. Coomarasamy. "Intrauterine Administration of Human Chorionic Gonadotropin (hCG) for Subfertile Women Undergoing Assisted Reproduction." *Cochrane Database of Systematic Reviews* 10, no. 10 (October 2018): article CD011537. http://doi.org/10.1002/14651858.CD011537.pub3.

Fanton, M., V. Nutting, F. Solano, P. Maeder-York, E. Hariton, O. Barash, L. Weckstein, D Sakkas, A. Copperman, and K. Loewke. "An Interpretable Machine Learning Model for Predicting the Optimal Day of Trigger during Ovarian Stimulation." *Fertility and Sterility* 118, no. 1 (July 1, 2022): 101–08, https://doi.org/10.1016/j.fertstert.2022.04.003.

Fauser, Bart C. J. M. "Towards the Global Coverage of a Unified Registry of IVF Outcomes." *Reproductive BioMedicine Online* 38, no. 2 (February 1, 2019): 133–37. https://doi.org/10.1016/j.rbmo.2018.12.001.

Glujovsky, D., C. Farquhar, A. M. Quinteiro Retamar, C. R. Alvarez Sedo, and D. Blake. "Cleavage Stage versus Blastocyst Stage Embryo Transfer in Assisted Reproductive Technology." *Cochrane Database of Systematic Reviews* 6 (June 2016): CD002118. https://doi.org/10.1002/14651858.CD002118.pub5.

"Gregory Pincus (1903–1967)." PBS. Accessed September 12, 2022. https://www.pbs.org/wgbh/americanexperience/features/gregory-pincus-1903-1967/.

Günther, V., S. von Otte, N. Maass, and I. Alkatout. "Endometrial 'Scratching': An Update and Overview of Current Research." *Journal of the Turkish German Gynecological Association* 21, no. 2 (June 2020): 124–29. https://doi.org/10.4274/jtgga.galenos.2020.2019.0175.

Heymann, D., L. Vidal, Y. Or, and Z. Shoham. "Hyaluronic Acid in Embryo Transfer Media for Assisted Reproductive Technologies." *Cochrane Database of Systematic Reviews* 9, no. 9 (September 2020): article CD007421. https://doi.org/10.1002/14651858.CD007421.pub4.

Hipp, H. S., S. Crawford, S. Boulet, J. Toner, A. A. E. Sparks, and J. F. Kawwass. "Trends and Outcomes for Preimplantation Genetic Testing in the United States." *JAMA* 327, no. 13 (April 5, 2022): 1288–90. http://doi.org/10.1001/jama.2022.1892.

"Intracytoplasmic Sperm Injection (ICSI) for Non-Male Factor Indications: A Committee Opinion." *Fertility and Sterility* 114, no. 2 (August 1, 2020): 239–45. https://doi.org/10.1016/j.fertnstert.2020.05.032.

Klitzman, R. "Deciding How Many Embryos to Transfer: Ongoing Challenges and Dilemmas." *Reproductive Biomedicine & Society Online* 3 (December 2016): 1–15. https://doi.org/10.1016/j.rbms.2016.07.001.

Lobo, I. "Pleiotropy: One Gene Can Affect Multiple Traits." *Nature Education* 1, no. 1 (2008): 10.

Maganto Pavón, E. "[Henry IV of Castilla (1454–1474)] An Exceptional Urologic Patient. An Endocrinopathy Causing the Uro-Andrological Problems of the Monarch. Impotence and Penile Malformation." *Archivos Espanoles de Urologia* 56, no. 3 (April 2003): 233–41.

Morshedi, M., H. E. Duran, S. Taylor, and S. Oehninger. "Efficacy and Pregnancy Outcome of Two Methods of Semen Preparation for Intrauterine Insemination: A Prospective Randomized Study." *Fertility and Sterility* 79, supp. 3 (June 2003): 1625–32. https://doi.org/10.1016/S0015-0282(03)00250-4.

Ombelet, W., and J. Van Robays. "Artificial Insemination History: Hurdles and Milestones." *Facts, Views & Vision* 7, no. 2 (2015): 137–43.

Sarwari, M., K. Beilby, K. Hammarberg, M. Hickey, and S. Lensen. "Endometrial Scratching in Australia, New Zealand and the United Kingdom (UK): A Follow-up Survey." *Human Fertility.* December 2021. http://doi.org/10.1080/14647273.2021.1995902.

"Scientists Say They Can Read Nearly the Whole Genome of an IVF-Created Embryo." *Science.* March 21, 2022. https://www.science.org/content/article/scientists-say-they-can-read-nearly-whole-genome-ivf-created-embryo.

Shi, Y., Y. Sun, C. Hao, H. Zhang, D. Wei, Y. Zhang, Y.Zhu, X. Deng, X. Qi, H. Li, et al. "Transfer of Fresh versus Frozen Embryos in Ovulatory Women." *New England Journal of Medicine* 378 (January 2018): 126–36. https://doi.org/10.1056/NEJMoa1705334.

Tharasanit, T., and P. Thuwanut. "Oocyte Cryopreservation in Domestic Animals and Humans: Principles, Techniques and Updated Outcomes." *Animals* 11, no. 10 (October 2021): 2949. https://doi.org/10.3390/ani11102949.

"The Alarming Rise of Complex Genetic Testing in Human Embryo Selection." *Nature*. March 21, 2022. https://www.nature.com/articles/d41586-022-00787-z.

Tšuiko, O., T. Jatsenko, L. K. P. Grace, A. Kurg, J. R. Vermeesch, F. Lanner, S. Altmäe, and A. Salumets. "A Speculative Outlook on Embryonic Aneuploidy: Can Molecular Pathways Be Involved?" *Developmental Biology* 447, no. 1 (March 2019): 3–13. https://doi.org/10.1016/j.ydbio.2018.01.014.

Weigel, G., U. Ranji, M. Long, and A. Salganicoff. "Coverage and Use of Fertility Services in the US." Kaiser Family Foundation. September 15, 2020. https://www.kff.org/womens-health-policy/issue-brief/coverage-and-use-of-fertility-services-in-the-u-s/.

Whyte, S., B. Torgler, and K. L. Harrison. "What Women Want in their Sperm Donor: A Study of More Than 1000 Women's Sperm Donor Selections." *Economics & Human Biology* 23 (December 2016): 1–9. https://doi.org/10.1016/j.ehb.2016.06.001.

Wilkinson, J., P. Malpas, K. Hammarberg, P. Mahoney Tsigdinos, S. Lensen, E. Jackson, J. Harper, and B. W. Mol. "Do à la Carte Menus Serve Infertility Patients? The Ethics and Regulation of In Vitro Fertility Add-ons." *Fertility and Sterility* 112, no. 6 (December 2019): 973–77. https://doi.org/10.1016/j.fertnstert.2019.09.028.

Viotti, M., A. R. Victor, F. L. Barnes, C. G. Zouves, A. G. Besser, J. A. Grifo, E.-H. Cheng, M.-S. Lee, J. A. Horcajadas, L. Corti, et al. "Using Outcome Data from One Thousand Mosaic Embryo Transfers to Formulate an Embryo Ranking System for Clinical Use." *Fertility and Sterility* 115, no. 5 (May 1, 2021): 1212–24. https://doi.org/10.1016/j.fertnstert.2020.11.041.

Xu, Z., W. Chen, C. Chen, Y. Xiao, and X. Chen. "Effect of Intrauterine Injection of Human Chorionic Gonadotropin Before Frozen-Thawed Embryo Transfer on Pregnancy Outcomes in Women with Endometriosis." *Journal of International Medical Research* 47, no. 7 (July 2019): 2873–80. https://doi.org/10.1177/0300060519848928.

INDEX

ABOUT THE AUTHOR

LESLIE SCHROCK is a founder, investor, and adviser to some of the top companies in health and technology. She is also the author of *Bumpin': The Modern Guide to Pregnancy*. Leslie was named one of the Most Creative People in Business by *Fast Company*, and her work has been featured in publications including the *Economist, Fortune, GQ*, and the *New York Times*, as well as on NPR and CNBC. She lives in Brooklyn with her husband and two sons.